HOTBODY.101

An Easy Diet & Exercise Program to Help You
Get Your Hot Body in 8 to 10 Weeks

Includes:

Easy to Do Workouts

An Easy to Understand Eating Program

Easy to Prepare Recipes

Developed by

Michael S. Kamins

NESTA Certified Personal Trainer
Professional Member, National Strength and Conditioning Association
and healthy survivor of college

*Developed for the college student who wants to combat "Freshman Fifteen" or
look "hot" for spring break – but works just fine for anyone who wants
to look good for vacation or a special event – even if it's just looking
and feeling good every day.*

First published by AuthorHouse 08/24/04

ISBN: 1-4184-1731-9 (sc)

Library of Congress Control Number: 2004090714

Printed in the United States of America
Bloomington, Indiana

This book is printed on acid-free paper.

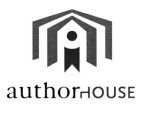

authorHOUSE

1663 LIBERTY DRIVE
BLOOMINGTON, INDIANA 47403
(800) 839-8640
www.authorhouse.com

Acknowledgements and Credits

If you've never written or tried to publish a book, you can't even guess what a production (literally) it really is. I wrote most of this program in about two weeks and after about a month of revising, I thought I was a step away from getting it on the shelf. Not a chance. Truth is, this is a better product because of the time many people took to read, comment and help me refine it. I would like to take some space to thank them, and also to say thanks to a few people who have helped shape and mold my ideas and goals, leading directly to the product you see in front of you. That's going to be a few years of people, so I know I won't be able to name them all (so if you do not see your name here, please know that I am grateful for any help you have been).

My parents and brother were the three people to whom I first confided the idea of helping college kids get in shape and they pushed me to actually sit down and write a book! For that I am truly grateful. Their ideas (often better than my own) helped me to fully complete this daunting task of writing a book. My parents went many steps further . . . underwriting this "project" and serving as sounding boards and editors. I'm going to just say "thanks," and I know you know all that I mean by that single word.

Outside of this inner circle are the only others who knew about the project and also gave insight and advice. They are two of my closest friends, Rami and Sarah, who gave both inspiration and support. Rami, who himself made a great change in his physique, was on many days my driving force to continue to go the gym. He is and will always be the best training partner I could have. Sarah listened for what amounted to many, many hours of frustration and venting, often times by phone, since she was at Providence College in Rhode Island while I was in school in Baltimore. Her patient ear and encouragement kept me going. You both have my sincere thanks.

The photographs were taken by Bill Geiger (Bill Geiger Photography, William K. Geiger, Washington, DC / www.billgeigerphoto.com.) Bill did a great job with the photos. He was more than happy to adjust his schedule as needed and extended other courtesies, for which I am deeply thankful. Even more than that, his enthusiasm for the project convinced me that this was definitely worth doing. He is a photographer of the finest quality, with many spectacular credits to his name. I hope this book is one you are proud to add to your list. Many thanks, Bill.

Thanks to the folks at Leisure Fitness in Rockville, Maryland – especially Jennifer, one of the store managers, for allowing us to set up and take most of the photos in her store using Leisure Fitness equipment. If you are interested in outfitting your own home gym, Leisure Fitness is a great place to start! In the DC metro area, come to the Rockville store and ask for Jennifer – she'll give you great assistance with your fitness goals.

I owe thanks also to Courtney Seymour, who I tracked down outside our gym in the pouring rain to ask her to pose for the lifting pictures. No doubt she thought I was crazy. Well, the pictures turned out great and I appreciate your willingness to take part in this endeavor.

Lastly I would like to acknowledge my many college friends with whom I partied, acted immature, loved, did flat out dumb things, and some smart things too, and basically grew with as a person. They are (but are definitely not limited to) Eric, Puma, Arden, Meredith, Jaime, Lauren, Lil' Kristen (I know these girls as the Loblolly girls), Ryan, Dorsey, Heather, Pence, Pete K, Pete Too, Mike S., Jean, Adam, and all the rest of the crew . . .

Dedication

For Nana and Grandma Milo, who believe that their grandchildren are meant to do great things.

For my surrogate uncle, Uncle Harry – I miss your humor, laughter and support. There will always be a place in my heart for "Chicken Bucket". Rest peacefully. I love ya.

Author's Notes

This book was written for you. That's right it is and was made for you! You will see and feel the amazing transformation that changing your body brings – both mental, and physical. Turn your own doubts into confidence! You have the ability, and now you have the tools, so no more excuses. Good luck, and just know if I can do it, then you definitely can too.

Disclaimer

HotBody.101 Diet and Exercise Program provides information about nutrition and physical activity that have been a successful approach to fitness for the author and others with whom he has worked. The materials contained here are not intended to be used for the diagnosis or treatment of a health problem or as a substitute for consulting a licensed health professional. References are included for informational use only.

Contents

Preface

*First, say to yourself what you would be; and then
do what you have to do. – Epictetus*

I want to share with you how I was able to get out of undergraduate school with a **HotBody**, and actually feeling <u>better</u> than when I got there. Undergrad – a time for experiencing everything you can get your mind around and your hands on – including (high on the list) take out food, pizza, beer and liquor. If you are currently in or have ever done college, you know this is always the "want" (to look good – no, look great) but most of the time kids are going in the other direction. Freshman fifteen (pounds you put on) can make you look pretty "snacky" by your junior year.

> **Not an undergrad?**
> **Not a problem.** The HotBody.101 Diet & Exercise Program has been a winner for all who have tried it– some are in their twenties, some in their fifties! Please read this preface – it gives some important info and provides a perspective.

I'm here to say that you can live the college life AND look great! Have your cake and eat it too, so to speak. In about 8-10 weeks, you can *look hot* for spring break or your beach vacation, or your cruise, or just for yourself . . . whatever. I'll simplify and clearly describe what to do – how to do the food and exercise – but first . . . I need to preface everything with a few clear statements.

I am a certified personal trainer (I earned this certification while an undergrad). I know my fair share about nutrition and exercise, body composition analysis, training and conditioning for specific goals and sports, and strength and aerobics training. My first responsibility to you is the same as it is to anyone I train - to advise you that, as with any program of exercise and diet, you need to be sure you are healthy enough to handle it! Get a general physical exam, just as you would if you were participating in a collegiate or intramural sport.

I am not a physician or a dietician. I am sharing with you what has worked for me as well as my clients, and what I've learned through my training and by reading many of the most knowledgeable professionals in the field.

I do not advocate binge drinking – period. I do, however, know what college is like, being that I am fresh out of undergrad and now in my first year of grad school. So I have designed my diet portion of the program to include moderate drinking (and "fat meals"). I hope you will take to heart the suggestions I have provided and use them wisely.

Books about exercise and wellness often present programs without considering real life situations. The goal, of course, is to sell the book. I have the same goal – to sell my book – but I have to be true to my experience and with the reality of college life.

Lots of things change when you go to college. You become independent. You have no curfew except your own. You eat lots, party lots, and may be influenced to drink lots.

For obvious reasons, drinking is counterproductive to nutrition, weight loss, and wellness. Many of these reasons are explained in detail throughout this book.

However, there are some other things that you should understand up front. I do not advocate drinking irresponsibly. Alcohol negatively influences good judgment. Excessive alcohol use lowers inhibitions. Under the influence you will do things you would never consider when not drinking. Some of these things have serious consequences.

Having said all that, in this book I will share with you my experience with alcohol as a college student. It is honest, direct, and did happen. I chose to be in charge of alcohol, not let drinking control me. You will have to do this for yourself. This holds true for any and all who choose to do this program, not just college students.

Finally, if you drink, know going into it you will have lowered your resistance to other, potentially negative influences. If you drink – don't drive! Read the box below. These facts are real!

According to the National Institute on Alcohol Abuse and Alcoholism, irresponsible and excessive drinking can result in:

- **Death** – clearly not a good thing. You jeopardize your own personal safety and that of others.
- **Injury** – Half-million students between the ages of 18 and 24 are unintentionally injured after drinking.
- **Assault** – Tons of students get into conflicts and fights more frequently with students after they have been drinking.
- **Sexual Abuse** – Instances of sexual abuse (date rape and sexual assault) increase dramatically as a result of alcohol consumption.
- **Unsafe Sex** – Increases in unprotected or coercive sex occur under the influence of alcohol.
- **Academic Problems** – Your grades may fall, next day hangovers will influence you to skip classes, and the further behind you get the more dropping out of school seems like a good alternative.
- **Health Problems/Suicide Attempts** – Physical ailments may increase as a result of alcohol, depression can occur, and depression has been linked with suicide.
- **Drunk Driving** – Not much to say here, except, if you drink please do not drive.
- **Vandalism/Property Damage** – Lots of college kids reveal that they have vandalized or damaged property while under the influence of alcohol.
- **Police Involvement** – This is a no-brainer. Review the list and you will see that the risks of legal action relate directly to lots of the above.
- **Dependency** – Early excessive alcohol abuse correlates with later-life alcohol dependency. Alcohol dependence is a life-long health risk. Why risk it?

That being said, this program worked for me. It has worked for all who have tried it. There is no reason that this diet and exercise program should not work for you. (To get a better idea, you may want to flip to Chapter 10 for FAQs.) I've designed this program for the average person with the idea of living the college life (or any busy life – young or old) but still getting into your best shape, much as I did. You too can achieve your desired results, but you have to stick to the nutritional and exercise options. I have found that when given an inch, many people try to take a mile. This can not work when using this program.

I'm excited to have this opportunity to help you achieve your goals, and congratulate you on beginning your journey towards a *HotBody*, a summer body, or just a body that you can be proud of. I'd wish you luck, but frankly you don't need it. ***Everything you need is now at your finger tips.***

Michael Kamins
May 2004

Chapter 1

Freshman Fifteen:
Setting A Tone

Success is getting what you want; happiness is wanting what you get.
– Dale Carnegie

Undergrad Rap

Cheeseburgers, pizza, tacos, fried foods . . . college cafeterias (and in the work place) run the gambit of foods that are fast, really tasty, and simply not nutritious. If you don't take your food choices seriously, you probably won't be eating foods that will help you achieve a Hot Body. You have to begin by becoming informed. No one is born knowing what foods to eat, and what exercises to do to achieve a beneficial level of fitness. I remember well being bombarded with the seemingly limitless array of "tasty" meals and "free" second helpings. Ultimately, I gained a good forty pounds in just my freshman year. Besides the negative affects this added weight had on my health, it also created for me a mindset of despair. It's a cycle that "feeds" on itself.

As my weight increased my drive to do something about it decreased. As I continued to get heavier and heavier, my self-esteem and confidence dipped and dipped. Little did I know at the time that other kids were having the same experience in college. I was only thinking about me and my own battle with the "Freshman Fifteen".

> **Not an undergrad?**
>
> Not a problem. If you have fairly recently been an undergrad, you may want to read this entire chapter to reminisce. If you are a parent of an undergrad, it might make you remember your own younger years. The object of this chapter is to give you an idea of where I was (and you may be too) – which also gives you an idea of where I was able to go (and you can too).

A little about me…

I went away to college as a two-sport star, or so I thought. Well, after a few weeks of school, my athletic present became my athletic past, and I settled into the life of not playing a competitive sport. Gradually I began to stay up later, eat more junk food (the ever-present vending machines), and exercise less and less. When I did do some exercise it was a half hearted attempt which usually ended up being bench presses and bicep curls. These two exercises seem to be the favorite of 90 percent of the gym goers in college.

To my dismay at the time, I was not achieving any results. The pressures of college – relationships, eating, studying, socializing, and plainly just fitting in – consumed my days and nights, and I hit rock bottom at 230 pounds. My "freshman fifteen" turned into a freshman forty, and I was in danger of continuing in that same direction. I believe I was borderline depressed. I hated being at school and came home every weekend. My inspiration came in the form of a negative comment by a friend I had not seen since my senior year.

As I sat in the stands at my high school's homecoming football game, I was approached by this guy and we exchanged hellos. During the conversation he made a passing comment that went exactly like this. "Man, they must have some good food at college, because you are getting big! Guess you're not playing a sport anymore, huh?" I just about cried. I smiled my way through it, successfully masking the pain that I felt inside. Interestingly enough, the only thing that I thought would make me feel better was food. You see, I began to eat for comfort and to mask my shame. Only now do I know that this is an all too common response. Needless to say, I left the game right away and found my way to a 7-Eleven.

As I walked in looking for those oh so comforting Reese's Peanut Butter Cups, I happened to glance at the magazines on the shelf. It was at that point that I saw them - those fit guys that covered the shelf on magazines like Men's Health, Men's Fitness, and Muscle and Fitness. I sat there thinking (with the peanut butter cups in my hand) that those guys on the covers were no different than me. Inside I was one of them, but on the outside I looked not even remotely close. It was at that moment that I decided I would take hold of life, and my fitness level and would one day appear on the cover of one of these magazines. As for the peanut butter cups, I left them sitting right there on the shelf, next to the guys I admired.

Start slowly . . . but start!

I began very slowly by jogging half a mile to a mile a day, and I joined the neighborhood Powerhouse Gym. A month into it I had lost about 5 pounds but was still not achieving the results I wanted in the time period I felt appropriate. It was then that I decided to take my next step. I chose to read anything and everything I could get my hands on. I read every magazine in print on the shelves, I read my roommates books from gym class, I read every single diet and exercise book out there at the time, and finally I decided that I would become certified in personal training. I told myself, that if I was certified in training then I couldn't let myself fall out of shape or else I would become not only discredited, but also the laughingstock of personal trainers.

Thus began my journey. I learned the proper movements and names of exercises, and I further educated myself on nutrition and diet. I hungered for information like I used to hunger for peanut butter cups. I started to devise a program for eating and exercising (the same one you will see on the accompanying pages) that would allow me to reach my goals in two months and also live a college life. I created menus from the foods that I knew the cafeteria had. I began to challenge myself to "eat clean" for up to 3 days at a time, and then up to five days at a time.

Along the way, I noticed something happening inside me. I was becoming more and more confident in myself everyday. I was my own best friend and partner in this process and had only myself to answer to when I strayed from the path. I began to see the definition that I had always wanted, but never had. All the while, I had the 8 o'clock morning classes, and went to the late night parties that go hand in hand with being an undergraduate in college. College is a time in your life like no other. (You begin to discover just how unique it is the minute you leave it, but that's another story). You really can make of it what you want. It is possible to live the college life and come out healthy, fit, cut and just feeling good about yourself. You can even partake in the events that make college, *college*.

The best thing about this plan is that it allows you the option to make mistakes. I made tons of mistakes. No one is perfect and no one should hold him/herself to that standard. You will be able to incorporate sensible drinking and junk food into this program and still achieve the results that you want! This program is all about making smart choices, the first one being choosing to do it. Best of all it works for anyone, not just undergrads.

Undergraduates are a lot like 9-to-5ers. We are all busy! Not everyone has the time to sit down and make intricate meals, and do hours on end of aerobic and strength training exercises. That is why this program is so effective for any and all who live life on the move. It is quick, easy, and user friendly. It is the one program that takes into account the time needs and pressures that college kids (and busy workers) have in their lives.

I want to thank you for choosing to do the program, and I want to congratulate you for taking that oh so crucial step towards achieving your very own Hot Body. A Hot Body, which is all of your doing! You will have no one to thank in 8 weeks, but yourself. All you need is now right here in front of you. Please allow yourself to take full advantage of your own amazing (you'll see) abilities . . .

Chapter 2

The Basics:
My 20 Basic Strategies

A journey of a thousand miles begins with one step. – Lao-tse

These twenty basics are the building blocks for achieving your **HotBody** – they are the foundation of your **HotBody.101 Diet and Exercise Program**.

1. **Eating Frequency** = at least 6 times a day, spaced out every two to three hours.

2. **Get your body fat tested** if you can. Go to any "chain" gym, or go online and order body fat calipers (about $10). I know this is going to be somewhat embarrassing - it sure as hell was for me - but just think about how you're going to feel with visible abs. (I do not believe in testing your weight to see fat loss results. Weight loss can be muscle loss as well. That is why I opt for the body fat percentage - and the mirror. The mirror being the best tool of all.)

3. **64 ounces of water a day** . . . a MUST . . . and this is the minimum.

4. **Simple meal management.** At each of the first 3 meals, include a portion of carbs and protein. Try to limit amount of carbohydrate intake for your last 3 meals. Vegetables can be eaten with any meal as they are free foods. (Basically eat more carbs early, less carbs late.)

5. **Eat good fats and limit saturated fats.** Good fats consist of unsaturated fats . . . CLA or flax seed oil are great options if you want to supplement your diet. Use PAM nonfat cooking spray (or a similar cooking spray) or olive oil. Fish (especially salmon) is a great way to get good fats into your diet.

6. **Snack on healthy LOW calorie options** . . . vegetables, dammit! This doesn't have to suck. Celery lined with a teaspoon of natural peanut butter actually tastes good!

7. **Active (but not SO hard) cardio every other day** . . . see the cardio section for a breakdown

8. **Choose an 8-week or 10-week plan** –

    - 8 Week Plan – Lifting 5 days a week
    - 10 Week Plan – Lifting 3 days a week

9. **Lift faithfully, according to your plan** . . . lifting might sound scary, but you are in and out of the gym in 60 minutes (8 week plan) or about 45 minutes (10 week plan) and it's more <u>fun</u> than you think . . . recruit a friend to be your partner . . . Believe it or not you will most likely feel energized and just plain better after your lifting sessions. Remember while you are busting your ass, others are eating fried foods and watching day time T.V. Guess who will have the better body!

10. **Supplement your diet appropriately.** Supplementation is anytime you put anything other than whole food into your diet. I AM NOT A DOCTOR. Please speak with a physician if you want to take anything other than water, protein (bars or mixes), good fats and a multivitamin.

11. **Seven (7) hours of sleep is a must**, no ifs, ands or buts. Take advantage of naps!

12. **Protein** – at least .75 to 1 gram of protein a day per pound of body weight will insure adequate muscle growth. This has worked well for me, my roommates, and anyone that I have trained. (This includes girls too! You girls need muscle to help burn fat. You see, the more lean muscle mass you have, the less fat you will carry!)

13. **Form is foremost!** The amount of weight you lift means nothing if you are not using correct form. Many times lifters can't lift as much correctly as they can with incorrect form. Don't be that person.

14. **Carbs are not the enemy!** You need carbs. Please don't cut them too low. Especially in college, when you need your brain to be working, carbs fuel your brain, so be smart and eat correctly. The amount of carbohydrates must stay above half of your body weight whether you do this program or not! Carbs fuel your brain, and you need all your brain power in college.

15. **Nutrition will constitute 70 percent of your program**. The other 30 will be spread out between belief, cardio, and weightlifting. So, as you might have guessed, mess up in nutrition and your goals will take a severe hit. I would rather skip a cardio or lifting session than a nutritious meal.

16. **Believe!** Believing in yourself is huge for the program to succeed. There will no doubt be people who won't think you can do it, and even more likely, simply don't want to change just because you do. SO – they may try to goad you into going along with them on a food run you don't want to do, just because they want your company. They are not invested in changing your body – that's your job. Believe in yourself - you can get those abs!

17. **Alcohol Facts.** A shot of Liquor, Gin, Rum, or Vodka is 109 calories. A regular beer is about 155 calories and 13 carbs. An average light beer is about 105 calories and 5 carbs. (This goes for "low carb" beer too.) Keep that in mind because excess calories will lead to fat storage. Now I know, I know - you don't count calories in my program (although I do keep track of them by writing them down), but you should know that these calories are the worst kind, and overindulgence will lead to fat retention.

18. **Be prepared!** Always be prepared with a food item that is nutritious, no matter where you go. Plan ahead. I carry nutrition bars in my car and book bag always. You should, too. Don't settle for a MilkyWay when you could have planned ahead and had a better option.

19. **Meal replacement drinks and bars** are definitely included in my program, if you can afford them. I think very highly of a few drinks and bars that I will mention in Chapter 4. I usually have a shake and a bar each day to replace two of my meals. These meal replacements allow me to be precise in the protein-to-carb ratio and give me a good satiated feeling after I eat or drink them. However, you definitely do not have to use them on this program. (Tip: protein causes you to get full quicker, and stay full longer.)

20. **Keep a food journal.** This is not a big deal! I repeat, this is SO NOT a big deal! Try it for a day and you will see how ridiculously easy this is, and believe me, those around you will start asking about it and thus give you credit for actually being somewhat organized! Basically you will write down everything you eat and drink. You will write down the carbs and protein counts. Trust me, it won't be difficult once you get started. (See Chapter 4.) Also, keep in mind that in making this plan user friendly, I have included calorie, carbohydrate, and protein counts for all foods on the food guide, so there is no guesswork or difficulty, only simplicity! (Vegetables are free foods, so they will not count towards and carbs, protein, or calories at all. We will talk about free foods in the diet section.)

Chapter 3

How to Eat At College:
Cafeteria and Take-Out Strategies

It's not that some people have willpower and some don't. It's that some people are ready to change and others are not. – James Gordon, M.D.

CAFETERIA
(or "The Commons," As I Knew It)

I loved "The Commons" once I got over my initial feeling of not wanting to walk the 74 steps it took to get there. Yeah, I was pretty lazy. Now not all cafeterias are laid out the same, and they sure as hell don't all serve the same food, but in this section I will lay out what to avoid and what to eat in order to make your university dining experience not only good for you, but appetizing as well.

Word to the wise, just because you can go back and get as much as you want does NOT mean you should! Portion size and moderation do mean something. They can mean the difference between your **HotBody** and not. Become aware of portion size by either reading the nutritional profile on an item, or using my method, which is to measure it against your clenched fist. One last thing, when choosing a portion size or fruit or a chicken breast, choose one piece! That is a portion size – not two apples and a pear . . . that would be three. (Yup, I passed statistics, although just barely.)

Know What You Are Eating!
Your ability to get good food is based on your knowledge of how to navigate the various sections of the cafeteria. I'll use "The Commons" of Salisbury University as the example of a standard buffet style set up, since that's popular everywhere these days. "The Commons" had a fried section (right when you walk in of course!), and also located next to the fruit. How smart is this? Anyone smelling the fried foods and or seeing them is going to breeze right by the fruit. (Sorry, but it's true.) Then there's a rotisserie section, a pasta section, a grilling section (burgers and such), a stir fry section, a pizza section, a bagel and cereal section, a deli section, and a salad bar and fruit area.

As far as the drinks go, I will talk about that at the end of the section, BUT that does not mean you should skip it or pay it little mind. Drinking extra calories and sugars will cancel your results (especially if you are planning on drinking other kinds of beverages at a party later.)

And, no, I haven't forgotten the dessert section – I am simply not going to address it because unless it is your fat meal, you need to pass this section over. A better choice would be eating at the cafeteria and then going back to the dorm or house or whatever you live in and having sugar free Jell-O or a sugar free popsicle (the fudge ones are good – no kidding).

OR, you can have a piece of fruit as dessert! You laugh, but fruit and vegetables are fabulous choices for anyone looking to shed pounds and fit into a bikini. Now, fruit is a little different than vegetables in that you need to limit yourself to one piece at a sitting since the sugar in fruit can be converted to fat.

The Buffet Guided Tour

OK, so here we go . . . this is your guided tour of the caf. (or <u>any</u> buffet). (See Chapter 4 for the actual Diet Plan.) I'm gonna take you through the cafeteria and we (you and I) are going to grab us some good tasting nutritious meals. So we walk in and right away smell the fried section. SKIP IT! Not only will it make you fat, it also will increase your bad cholesterol promote overall bad health and make you feel sluggish, SKIP IT!

OK, good job! Now, on to the **rotisserie section**. Now, in your caf. this might amount to some chicken or turkey dish that is not even remotely appetizing. If this is so then just skip it. BUT, if this is the place where you find the slicing station, then we must take a closer look. What we are looking for is a nice clean relatively low fat cut of meat (protein). So any cut that is listed on the food guide is doable here, just be wary of portion size.

Often times, these stations have steamed vegetables, and some kind of potatoes. Vegetables are always great! Potatoes are also great choices for your carbohydrate portion of the meal. (I like the nutritional value of yams, sweet potatoes, or red skin potatoes, but really any baked or boiled potato is better than fries, chips etc.)

So, if you have a lean cut of meat and a potato with some vegetables, you have yourself a great meal! Basically you are done. I know there are many more choices but remember, on this program, portion size and moderation are the keys. (Nutrition is 70 percent of the plan!!!)

Now that I have said that, you are always welcome to have at it at the **salad bar**. (Many of the items you will find here are free foods!) Stay away from any regular dressing, and choose lighter versions if you have to have any at all. Also, if you are choosing oil and vinegar, (which is by far the best dressing nutritionally), go easy on the oil and heavy on the vinegar for taste. A tip at the salad bar is to always carry two plates or bowls, one for the salad and one for the dressing. Use the dip technique so you can regulate the amount of dressing. Do not drench your salad with any kind of dressing, even light (vinegar excluded, cause the nutritional profile is excellent), because you are only adding excess calories that will be converted to fat.

OK, so we conquered the rotisserie section and the salad bar. Let's move on to the **Pasta** area. Oh boy, pasta. You are going to hate this, but this is a diet killer. No one eats one serving of pasta, let alone eats it plain. So it is my suggestion to skip this section altogether. Use pasta sparingly and ONLY if it's wheat or low carb. (These pastas can be ordered on the internet, and are pretty good!). However, I don't imagine school cafeterias provide this. You will need to go without normal pasta for the next 8 to 10 weeks if you want the bikini or to be comfortable shirtless. Hey, everyone makes sacrifices . . . this is a small one!

Next up, oh boy, the **grilling section**. This section is either the best place you can be, or the worst. Choose the burger and you are hurting your plan, let alone that food isn't on the food guide. But, choose the grilled chicken and you are well on your way to being HOT. Here is what I do, and what I suggest. Unless they have a wheat bread bun, or multigrain bun, ditch it. Plain white bread (along with plain white rice) is a no go. These carbohydrates will shoot your insulin level way up, causing you to <u>store fat</u>. So, take the grilled chicken and all the fixings (minus mayo) and put them in your salad. Voila - a good tasting chicken salad!

Always keep in mind if the caf. is offering a food that I have not mentioned here but is on the list, then go right ahead and enjoy, just practice portion control. For instance, many cafeterias offer a grilled fish option – this is also a great choice, as long as it's not cooked in butter! **Stir-fry**? Yup, I

> *A note about cheese:*
> I'm not a huge fan of cheese in my diet in the first place because of the high amounts of fat, and the fact that a little cheese equals a lot of calories. (Sucks, 'cause you know me and cheese fries.) Yet, I do think that it has a place, for instance, in your fat free omelets that you will learn how to cook (see recipes).

love me some stir-fry, dammit. Unfortunately, not many cafeterias are willing to stir fry with extra virgin olive oil. Let alone I would want them to use much less than the usual amount, so this is an area you want to skip, unless you in fact can use extra virgin olive oil or PAM cooking spray (like when you are cooking for yourself). If so, then dive right in to some chicken with mixed vegetables! (Remember, skip the white rice.)

The **pizza station** should be a <u>no brainer</u> for you by now. You don't need all that great tasting cheese and sauce bubbling up to utter perfection . . . damn . . . anyway you got to skip it if you are doing my plan. I know it sucks, but hey, that's why there is a fat meal! Knock yourself out during your fat meal, I sure as hell do.

Lastly, the **cereal and bagel section**. Hey, do me a favor and look at the food guide (next chapter). Are cereals and bagels on there? NO. So skip it, unless you can get plain old-fashioned oatmeal. This is the best carbohydrate in my book. I like the taste, and it is flat out awesome in giving you energy in the gym. (You can sweeten oatmeal with any of the artificial sweeteners, and fruit if you would like as well. Check out my oatmeal recipes in the back for other ways to make it doable.)

The **deli section** is also a good friend of mine. I love turkey sandwiches on wheat bread with any and all the fixings I can find that are on the food guide. Many diets say no to lunchmeats. I say go right ahead; you just have to make smart choices. Ask the server for the low fat or fat free cuts of meat. Healthy Choice makes great stuff, so does Dietz and Watson. Skip the roast beef, unless it's a very low fat version like Healthy Choice, and even then, practice moderation. All these meats will come in full fat versions. If that is all they serve, then skip it. But I am pretty sure most cafeterias will have a lower fat (low sodium is a plus too) version of lean sliced ham, turkey breast, and chicken breast. (Salami is a no. Nice try though.) Please feel free to add on a side salad to your sandwich, or make it a huge salad, I don't care. This is a definite good bet for your diet.

And now, the **drink section**. This can be a killer, but we aren't going to let that happen, right? See the sodas? SKIP them! Soda is sugar water, plain and simple and has no place in this program. However, I do allow diet soda, whereas other mainstream diets don't. This is my reasoning. Diet soda contains no sugar, and it has some taste. I mean come on, water isn't everyone's favorite drink. Here is the catch though; with each cup of diet soda comes a cup of water, got it? So you are making sure you are getting your daily fill of water. As far as fruit juices go, they are a NO. Fruit juice is also a lot like sugar water. Stick to real fruit (those listed on the food guide) and possibly the flavored waters or diet teas. (Fruit2o and Snapple make good tasting low or no calorie stuff. Gatorade's Propel water is good too, if you must have some taste.)

So did we do it?

I think we did. Feels good, huh? Hey, do me this quick favor. Look around you. You see everyone sitting down with their deep fat fried food, and sugary drink and desserts, and tell me how many of them are ripped, jacked, buff? Exactly my point. Good Job. (There will no doubt be one or two girls or guys who can eat whatever the hell they want and stay lean as shit and cut up all year . . . . Know what I say to them? "Good for you. I wish I had your genetics. Unfortunately I was born with fat man genetics." I can't eat that crap and stay lean, and I imagine neither can you since you are reading this book. So here we are with our healthy meals. Hey, there is power in numbers ☺)

Well, we have conquered one of the main obstacles in getting fit in college. *You versus the cafeteria*. Good for us. I won't lie to you and say everything we eat tastes fabulous, 'cause it doesn't – but it's not bad tasting, either. But I will tell you that when someone on the beach looks at your body and then makes eye contact and smiles, it feels damn good. As I've said many times . . . I know how you feel.

OK, all you vegetarians out there. You are thinking this guy has a good program, but it isn't for me. NOT TRUE! You can substitute my all time favorite supplement for any protein choice, that supplement being protein powder. There are many types of protein powder, take a look at my suggestions in the supplement section. So buy yourself some powder, and a shaker and bring it with you to meals. Shake up your protein and sip that with your salad, or other choice from the food guide! (See added help.) PLUS, there are many meat free high protein meal products located in your supermarket's freezer section. Try Boca Burgers ™ and all the different variations that they sell. Check the food guide for help in with meatless products. They have options like meatless hotdogs, meatless ground beef, meatless sausages, and all are good choices. Natural peanut butter can also play a role in this diet as long as you practice portion control. Add it to celery or with multi grain bread for a snack or a meal. Tofu can also be a good choice to add to any carbohydrate dish for a hit of protein. **(My dad, known as Bigz or Pop, is a vegetarian. Yet he lost a good 20 pounds and added a whole bunch of muscle. He also dropped his body fat significantly, all the while not eating any meat.)**

TAKE OUT / EAT OUT IDEAS

I don't expect you to sit home when everyone else is eating out! There are some pretty easy ways to make the nutritional part of the program work, even with take out or eating out.

- Choose restaurants that offer healthy choices based on the program diet.

- Collect menus from your favorite restaurants so you can plan your selections.

- Chicken Out, Boston Market and Subway offer options that work well with this diet. So do other restaurants, you just have to be wise and order according to the plan.

- Most restaurants offer some kind of grilled chicken of grilled chicken salad.

- A great meal is take out Chinese steamed chicken (or beef) and broccoli, sauce on the side.

- Don't arrive at the restaurant hungry as all hell. Eat something small before you go – like an apple, serving of fat free yogurt or vegetables.

- Ask your server to wrap half up before it's served (it can be another great meal, later!).

- Share an entrée with a friend.

- Stay away from buffets, or if you must go, choose wisely. Just because it's a buffet, does not mean you have to go back a billion times. Remember portion control.

- Don't fall victim to healthy-sounding foods, such as restaurant-made egg salad or chicken salad sandwiches. These options are often very high in fat and high-glycemic carbs.

- Order dressings, sauces and gravies on the side so you can practice the "dip technique." Don't eat more than half of the serving provided.

- Ask questions about how the food is prepared – "Is [the food] cooked in olive oil as opposed to butter?"

- Choose items that are served broiled, grilled, baked, roasted, poached or steamed.

- Substitute a side salad, baked potato or sweet potato in place of fries.

- If you order coffee drinks, request fat free (skim) milk.

RECAP - 10 MAIN POINTS

1) Skip the fried foods section. Period.

2) Choose lean cuts of meat over fatty cuts like prime rib.

   • Chicken breast or turkey breast is a great choice.

   • The sandwich section provides you with a lean cut of meat (protein choice) with a great carbohydrate option (wheat Bread, or multi-grain bread).

3) Cereal and bagels are a NO!

   • Flat out – there is no way to eat a portion size.

   • The nutritional value is just bad - so they stay a NO (except old fashioned oatmeal).

4) Skip the dessert section.

   • Substitute a piece of fruit if you must have something sweet (or try ½ of a protein bar)

   • Or go home and grab some sugar-free Jell-O or a "no sugar added" popsicle.

5) Stir-fry is a no-no, unless you can have the chef make the accommodations mentioned earlier.

6) Skip the pasta.

   • Pasta will lead to fat storage; there is no way around it.

   • Remember you want the looks on the beach, and it's only 8 (or 10) weeks!

7) Any type of grilled fish is a great choice!

   • Make sure it is grilled or boiled with minimal butter.

8) Use portion control and moderation.

   • Remember, this is just a meal.

   • So what if it is buffet style? That does not mean you need to eat everything in sight.

9) The salad bar is the place to be.

   • Be creative, make a salad and add a lean cut of meat.

10) Eat whatever you want during your fat meal.

   • Hit every section if you want - I don't care.

   • Have fun!

Chapter 4

HotBody Eating Program

Curious things, habits. People themselves never knew they had them. – Agatha Christie

First of all…you are allowed one fat meal a week, and one day that allows alcohol consumption, as long as you are of legal age and drink responsibly (see preface for the dangers of over consumption of alcohol). On your fat meal, I encourage you to go to town! Eat anything you want, and don't feel any shame or remorse. You have earned it, so enjoy your reward!

Moderation

The key to my diet is moderation. As the saying goes, everything in moderation - even moderation. (That's why I have a fat meal and allow the ability to drink.) I go by portion size at my meals. A portion size in my plan is the size of your fist. However, one chicken breast also is a portion size. Basically if you have a chicken breast, don't try to measure it against the size of your fist, just call it one portion. Just be smart, if the chicken breast is the size of your hand times three, then cut it in half and eat half now and half at your next meal. In order to make this eating plan even simpler, I have included a food chart that lists the carbohydrate, protein, and calorie count for EVERY food that is allowed in the program. Therefore, you won't have to guess, and filling out the food journal will be ridiculously easy. This also makes the ability to calculate your totals at the end of the day as easy as possible. You see, I told you this program is really simple. **Remember, you are allowed one day with alcohol, and one fat meal a week!**

Not an undergrad? Not a problem. This chapter presents an eating plan that is nutritional and easy to implement, once you get the hang of it, whether you're in school, at work, or at home.

Protein

Protein is a fat burning tool, bottom line. You have to eat at least .75 to a gram of protein for each pound you weigh to build muscle (girls too) . . . SO, let's use me as an example. I weigh 190 - so I need at the least 142.5 grams of protein a day. (.75 x 190 = 142.5). Pretty easy, huh? Protein is the building block of muscle and a speedy metabolism. Please see the following chart I have provided for your totals based on your body weight.

Carbohydrates

Carbohydrates are the absolute key to my eating program. Here's how I have been able to maximize muscle gain and minimize fat storage – rotating carbohydrate consumption. By rotating our carbohydrate consumption we will maximize our fat burning while minimizing our fat storing. I have developed an eating plan based on the "UP and DOWN" approach. It's so simple - it's almost so easy that everyone ought to know it already, hehehe, but let's let those other guys figure it out on there own.

- Monday, Wednesday, Friday, and Sunday (these are "UP" days) - your total carb intake will be your body weight plus 75. Using me as an example: I weigh 190, so 190 + 75 = 265 . . . 265 grams will be my total carbohydrate intake these days. (Keep in mind this is not an exact science. So if my goal is 265 and I turn out with 249, then that's fine. Same would be true if I end up with 278. Just try to stay within 15-20 grams of the recommended total for the day.)

- Tuesday, Thursday, and Saturday – (These are "DOWN" days) - your carbs will be equivalent to ¾ (.75) of your body weight. Using me as an example: 190 x .75 = 142 grams total carbohydrates for me these days. (Once again, just try to stay within 15-20 grams of the recommended amount.)

- One last thing about these wonderful carbs - do your best to eat them at least 2 hours before you go to sleep. A simple rule is "more carbs early, less carbs late."

Down/Up Day Chart by Body Weight

In continuing with the hope of making this program the easiest program around, I have provided for you, the carbs. that you should eat on either the "Up" day or the "Down" day. Just simply find your weight and scroll across. I also have provided your protein intake based on weight. I have gone every ten pounds, but if you fall in between, just use the weight below you. Keep in mind the protein category is your total you should get everyday.

Body Weight	Carb "Up" Day	Carb "Down" Day	Protein
lbs.	grams	grams	(any day) grams
110	185	82.5	82.5
120	195	90.0	90.0
130	205	97.5	97.5
140	215	105.0	105.0
150	225	112.5	112.5
160	235	120.0	120.0
170	245	127.5	127.5
180	255	135.0	135.0
190	265	142.5	142.5
200	275	150.0	150.0
210	285	157.5	157.5
220	295	165.0	165.0
230	305	172.5	172.5
240	315	180.0	180.0
250	325	187.5	187.5
260	335	195.0	195.0
270	345	202.5	202.5
280	355	210.0	210.0
290	365	217.5	217.5
300	375	225.0	225.0

Calories

This program does not call for you to count calories – although you can if you'd like. I have included the calorie count on my foods as well as on my food guide I provided just so I could show you how to keep them in check, but it is the CARBS and the PROTEIN I want you to pay attention too. All calories are not created the same however. Eating 200 calories of lean protein (chicken breast) and 200 calories of candy won't have the same impact, but would count the same. I have found that counting carbohydrates and protein is a much more useful way to regulate your ability to burn fat and build muscle on the program. Also, I do count how many meals I eat a day, and I use meal size and consistency. And, I do write down everything I eat and I suggest you do the same. Keeping a food (and drink) journal helps me keep on track and has a funny way of helping me not eat too much crap or drink too much.

The Journal

Now when I say you have to write it down, I mean you have to write <u>everything</u> down. Those three Miller Lights, yup! That shot of tequila, ummhmm. The only time you don't have to write down what you eat (although u still might want to) is on your fat meal. Eat whatever the hell ya want. I sure do. I'm partial to pizza and nearly any takeout food. Although cheese fries are right up there too, hehe. Anyway, during your fat meal feel free to have anything you would like. Do not however make your fat meal into a full fat day, where every meal is horrible, and then on top of this put down a rack of alcohol. Please don't ruin the gains that you have made. I have no problem with a fat meal, but not a fat day, and or a fat weekend. (See sample journals at end of chapter.)

Good vs. Bad Carbs

OK, so here we go with Good versus Bad carbs. (These are also known as high glycemic versus low glycemic, but this isn't a medical dictionary, so I'm going to call them good and bad.) Good carbs do not raise your insulin levels too high. The goal is to have your insulin stay steady, not fluctuate up or down. Good carbs are the ones that promote energy release (calories are an energy measure by the way) and bad carbs are the ones that store as fat. These definitions are subject to disagreement, but look, this is my food plan and I don't claim to be a bioscience major. We will try to eat all good carbs, except for the fat meal. (Please see the food guide for a list of good carbs. that are allowed, as well as lean protein choices.)

Portion Size and Moderation

Now I am more than sure there will be readers who disagree with my carb choices or have an opinion about them, but look – these worked for me and all those who I have trained, so I am comfortable saying they WILL work for you. The key here is portion size and moderation. The carbohydrate manipulation in this program actually will act as a fat burner! Yet, one sweet potato should not become two, or one bowl of oatmeal should not be three or four bowls. Likewise one chicken breast is not 3 chicken breasts. These extra calories will be stored as fat even if you are eating relatively clean food. (A note about egg whites: one portion = from 6 to 8 egg whites.)

Snack Foods to Avoid

Below I have noted a few snack foods that you might be thinking are excellent choices. Sorry, these foods are no no's unless it's a fat meal, and even then, you might want to choose a better fat meal (like cheese fries hehe . . .). You'll notice that none of these are on the food plan guide anyway, so the point is moot.

- Regular or reduced fat triscuits
- Rice Cakes
- Popcorn
- Chips
- Pretzels
- Any and all reduced fat lies that are out there

Dessert

Now don't think I've forgotten about the most important meal . . . DESSERT . . . there are many options for dessert. The goal here is for dessert to be low sugar if any at all, low calorie and tasting good. I have the worst sweet tooth ever, as anyone who knows me can confirm. So I have spent the good part of two years searching for good tasting desserts. My personal favorites are sugar free Jell-O (a free food), no sugar added and or sugar free popsicles or fudgcicles, or a no sugar fat free pudding, which Jell-O also makes. If you look at my food list, you will see a variety of dessert offerings that will help curb the sweet tooth and satiate hunger as well. Remember that these will also count towards your carb and protein intake, so choose wisely. Portion size is important, as always! Read the back of the label and see what a portion size is and then eat accordingly. Some good desserts . . .

- Sugar free or no sugar added popsicles or fudgcicles
- Sugar free Jell-O pudding (with skim milk)
- Sugar free Jell-O (a staple for me)
- Nutrition bar or shake (see A*dded Nutritional Help*, below)
- Apple, pear, orange or other fruit . . . try to eat these 2 hours before going to sleep though).

Water

Water is the lifeline of our diet. I need it, you need it, we all need it. You have to count your carbs. and protein in your journals, however I do not make you count water. Yet, it might be a good idea, especially since you need 64 ounces a day. 64 ounces is not a lot, despite what you might be thinking. It is actually quite easy to get this much water in a day. Bring a water bottle with you wherever you go. Going to class? Have the water bottle. Going to the movies? Bring a water bottle. You should always have a water bottle with you at the gym while performing either cardio or lifting. Sip it throughout the day, and before you know it you'll be taking in even more than 64 ounces! If there is one thing that the body needs more than anything, it is water, do not skimp on it! The best thing about water is that it actually makes you feel fuller. This means you <u>won't be hungry</u>, so drink up!

Added Help . . . Nutritional Bars and Such

OK, I want you to know that I have not been paid to endorse any of the products I will mention here. Although I choose to use these shakes or bars, it is up to you whether you include them in the actual plan. They simply provide for me a more convenient way to keep track of protein and carbs. As well as making sure I have healthy food available at all times. I just think they taste best. I have tried just about every protein or "total nutrition" bar on the market and I have my favorites. I am a strong believer in nutrition bars and shakes. I drink or eat at least one a day. Now consider – these <u>do</u> count towards your meal totals, but then again it's not like you're cheating by eating them, and some (believe it or not) really taste good.

The bars can, however, become expensive. There are some ways to minimize your expense. For example, GNC offers 20% percent off everything they sell for the first 7 days of every month, so go and buy your stuff then! If you like the bars and shakes – buy them in bulk. (Buy a box, not just one at a time.) You will save a lot of money that way. Vitamin Shoppe also is great for saving money. Often the same products are sold cheaper than in other nutritional stores, and you can earn points toward free purchases. Lastly, try ordering online. I personally use Netrition.com – the service is quick and the products have been fresh.

You should experiment to see which ones you like the best. I don't think there is a "best" bar or shake out there, but I do have my favorites. They are listed below, but here are some other options. (Please understand there are a billion of them, the ones I mention here are the ones I allow while doing to **HotBody.101** program)

- ***Luna Bars*** [not just for woman] (170 cals. 26 carbs. 10 grams protein – Toasted Nuts 'N Cranberry flavor)
- ***Balance Bars*** (200 cals. 22 carbs. 14 grams protein)
- ***Myoplex Carb Sense Bars*** (240 cals. 22 carbs. 30 grams protein – Apple Cinnamon flavor)
- ***Myoplex Shakes*** (280 cals. 24 carbs. 42 grams protein -Chocolate flavor)
- ***Pure Protein Bars*** (300 cals. 26 carbs. 32 grams protein – Blueberry Cheesecake flavor)

> ***Preparation tip -***
> Purchase a couple of "shakers containers" at your nutrition store. That's the handiest way to make the shakes. If you have a blender, it's a great way to make those shakes taste like a Baskin Robbins treat..

So what do I use? I list them below. You will see a lot of products made by Labrada. I really like this stuff, I can't say it enough. Their shakes and bars are the best, in my opinion, for achieving the goals this book sets out to accomplish. They offer such flavors as Kiwi-Strawberry, Chocolate Ice Cream, and Pina Coloda in shakes. They also offer a bar that is a snickers twin called Lean Body Gold (caramel peanut.)

- *Labrada Low Carb. (also called Carb Watchers) Lean Body Shakes* (230 cals. 12 carbs. 42 grams protein – all flavors)

- *Labrada Lean Body Gold bars* . . . these taste like eating a candy bar, but have an excellent nutritional profile. (300 cals, 30 carbs. 30 grams protein –Caramel Peanut flavor)

- *Labrada Lean Body Low Carb bars* (sometimes called **Carb Watchers**) . . . Also great tasting, lower in sugar (by a little) than the Gold version (260 cals. 18 carbs. 30 grams protein – Texas Pecan Pie flavor)

- *Nitro Tech bars* made by **Muscletech** . . . these are also very good tasting and pack a lot of protein into a bar with low carbs. (290 cals. 32 carbs. 35 grams protein – Strawberry Cheesecake flavor)

- *Optimum Pro Complex protein powder* . . . this is one of the main mixable proteins I use (the other being the Labrada shakes) and will stay that way. It has a mix of some great proteins in it and is instantly mixable. This is the protein powder I would recommend for anyone interested in using this kind of supplement. It tastes good, and is low in calories, carbs, fat and high in protein per serving. You can eat a carb rich meal and use this powder to up your protein. That's particularly helpful if you are a vegetarian. And both girls and guys can use protein powder to help build lean muscle.

Journal Samples –

These are samples of my daily food journal.* (I count calories too, but this is optional for you. Protein and carbs are most important in this diet, because that's what stokes your metabolism and helps you burn fat.)

This is a sample **"DOWN carb"** day on the UP-DOWN plan.

Time	Food (1 serving)	Carbs (grams)	Protein (grams)	Calories (optional)
9:30 am	Oatmeal (Old Fashioned)	30	5	150
	Scrambled cheese eggs (see recipes)	4	25	240
Noon	Grilled Chicken breast	N/A	30	290
	Cucumber (any vegetable)	Free	Free	Negligible
	No sugar added popsicle	10	0	50
2 pm	Protein bar	29	30	290
4:30 pm	Turkey breast sandwich on 2 slices whole wheat	34	30	350
	Fresh sliced peppers (any vegetable)	Free	Free	Negligible
6:30 pm	"Cafeteria grilled chicken salad" with balsamic vinegar (see recipes)	N/A	30	290
8:30 pm	Mike's spicy and cheesy egg white omelet (see recipes)	4	25	240
	Sugar-free Jell-O (any flavor)	Free	Free	Negligible
11 pm Optional	Labrada Protein shake	12	42	230
	TOTALS for the day	123	217	2130
This is MY food guide based on my weight and goals – yours won't look exactly like this. Yours will match YOUR weight and goals.				

This is a sample **"UP carb"** day on the high-low plan.

Time	Food (1 serving)	Carbs (grams)	Protein (grams)	Calories (optional)
9:30 am	Oatmeal	30	5	150
	Scrambled Cheese Eggs (see recipes)	4	25	240
Noon	Oatmeal (Old Fashioned)	30	5	150
	Turkey Burger (see recipes)	15	27	250
	(on wheat bread)	13	3	70
2 pm	Labrada Protein Shake	12	42	230
	Cucumber	n/a	n/a	n/a
	Apple	30	0	100
4:30 pm	Grilled Chicken Breast	n/a	30	290
	Sweet Potato	45	5	150
6:30 pm	Chicken Pita (Whole Wheat)	40	40	320
8:30 pm	Protein bar	29	30	290
	Fresh Sliced Pepper	n/a	n/a	n/a
	No sugar added popsicle	10	0	50
11 pm Optional	Scrambled Cheese Eggs (see recipes)	4	25	240
	TOTALS for the day	262	237	2430

Again, this is MY food guide based on my weight and goals – yours won't look exactly like this. Yours will match YOUR weight and goals.

Reading the Labels!
Since 1994 food manufacturers have been required by the Food and Drug Administration (FDA) to include food labels (or Nutrition Facts labels) on product packaging so that consumers have accurate nutritional information about the food they purchase. But food labels are more than just a federal requirement – once you understand the information they provide, you can use food labels as a guide to planning healthier meals and snacks. [From http://www.lifeclinic.com/focus/nutrition/]

Understanding Serving Sizes
Please pay attention to serving size indications on the box. Here is a sample food label. It shows everything we need to know. This label is Quaker Oats oatmeal. Be mindful of the protein and carbohydrate counts. If you happen to get mixed up with serving size, you always have the rule of thumb for the **HotBody.101** eating plan, which states that any serving of anything on the food guide is roughly the size of a clenched fist. If you want to measure it, great! But, if you don't have time then just go with the clenched fist rule. We can see here though that ½ cup oatmeal provides us with 27 carbohydrates, 5 grams of protein, and 150 calories. You see, it really is easy as pie! Well, maybe not pie, but you get the idea haha.

Nutrition Facts
Serving Size: ½ Cup dry (40g)
Servings Per Container 30

Amount Per Serving:
Calories	150
Calories from Fat	25

Total Fat 3g		5%
Saturated Fat .5g		2%
Polyunsaturated Fat 1g		
Monounsaturated Fat 1g		
Cholesterol 0mg		0%
Sodium 0mg		0%
Total Carb 27g		9%
Dietary Fiber 4g		15%
Soluble Fiber 2g		
Insoluble Fiber 2g		
Sugars 1g		
Protein 5g		

Vitamin A	0%
Vitamin C	0%
Calcium	0%
Iron	10%

Ingredients:
100% Natural Whole Grain
Quality Rolled Quaker Oats

Food Choices

Again, I've kept this to an easy to read, straightforward list to start. Please, I encourage you to try some of the easy recipes that are located in the back of the book. As you become familiar with the program's eating regimen, feel free to try all sorts of new recipes that include the foods on the food guide. If you do discover any great recipes, please send them along to me and I will definitely consider including them for future volumes of the book. And of course, I will give you the credit in the future volumes!

Main points to remember:

- One portion of protein and vegetables equals one meal.
- Add one portion of carbohydrates to at least three of the six meals. (Less carbs after roughly 8 p.m.)
- Vegetables can always be added at any time as snacks or if hunger still occurs.
- You can add condiments, if desired, such as fat free mayo (serving=1 teaspoons), mustard and ketchup (serving=1 teaspoons).

To get started, you can use a chart like my sample food journals. Just jot it down on notebook paper or use the programs Excel or Word if you are computer literate. It really doesn't have to be fancy. Just something so you can get into the habit of making the right food selections. Then you can simply select foods from the chart on the next page(s). I actually use a Five Star ™ notebook and just write it all down.

FOOD CHART

Food	Category	Calories	Protein	Carbs
Chicken Breast, Skinless (7 ounces)	Protein	290	30	0
Cottage Cheese, non-fat (1 cup)	Protein	85	15	5
Crab (6 ounces)	Protein	105	23	0
Deli, Sliced Chicken (6 ounces)	Protein	195	22	7
Deli, Sliced Ham (6 ounces)	Protein	205	20	7
Deli, Sliced Turkey (6 ounces)	Protein	200	25	5
Egg White (1) or equivalent substitute	Protein	20	5	0
Ground Beef, Extra Lean (6 ounces)	Protein	270	30	0
Haddock (1 medium fillet)	Protein	165	20	0
Lobster (6 ounces)	Protein	125	17	0
Orange Roughy (1 medium fillet)	Protein	180	25	0
Pork Tenderloin (lean) (6 ounces)	Protein	220	35	8
Salmon (1 medium fillet)	Protein	250	19	0
Shrimp (6 ounces)	Protein	105	23	0
Slice Fat Free Cheese	Protein	30	5	2
Steak, Flank (6 ounces)	Protein	290	40	0
Steak, Top Round (6 ounces)	Protein	300	40	0
Steak, Top Sirloin (6 ounces)	Protein	300	40	0
Swordfish (1 medium steak)	Protein	250	31	0
Tuna 3.25 oz can, in water	Protein	112	24	0
Tuna fresh (1 medium steak)	Protein	290	40	0
Turkey Breast, Skinless (7 ounces)	Protein	280	30	0
Turkey Burgers (see recipe)	Protein	250	27	15
Turkey Dogs (2 for a serving -store bought)	Protein	150	10	3
Turkey, Lean Ground (7 ounces)	Protein	230	40	0
Veggie burgers (Boca, Morningstar, etc)	Protein	80	12	7

Note: Protein will stand to be the building block of our gaining muscle, which in turn will cause us to burn more fat! You see, muscle burns more calories than fat, so if we increase our muscle, we decrease our fat and thus turn our bodies into fat burning furnaces. The same moderation concept holds true here too though. So just make sure that that one chicken breast does not become 2, and that the 8 ounces of flank steak does not become 16 ounces.

* With regards to meatless products, like Boca burgers and such, experiment with the different flavors. However Boca now has a pizza out, and it is not approved for this program. Stick to the burgers, chicken, hot dogs, ground beef, and breakfast sausages offered by Boca, and other meatless products. Read the labels as to the nutritional profile.

Michael S. Kamins

FOOD CHART

Food	Category	Calories	Protein	Carbs
Artichoke	Vegetable	free	free	free
Asparagus	Vegetable	free	free	free
Broccoli	Vegetable	free	free	free
Brussels Sprouts	Vegetable	free	free	free
Cabbage	Vegetable	free	free	free
Carrot	Vegetable	free	free	free
Cauliflower	Vegetable	free	free	free
Collard Greens	Vegetable	free	free	free
Corn	Vegetable	free	free	free
Cucumber	Vegetable	free	free	free
Eggplant	Vegetable	free	free	free
Green Beans	Vegetable	free	free	free
Green Pepper	Vegetable	free	free	free
Lettuce (Iceberg)	Vegetable	free	free	free
Lettuce (Romaine)	Vegetable	free	free	free
Lettuce (Other)	Vegetable	free	free	free
Mushrooms	Vegetable	free	free	free
Onion	Vegetable	free	free	free
Peas	Vegetable	free	free	free
Red Pepper	Vegetable	free	free	free
Spinach	Vegetable	free	free	free
Tomato	Vegetable	free	free	free
Yellow Pepper	Vegetable	free	free	free
Zucchini	Vegetable	free	free	free

Note: Vegetables are what we will consider *free* foods, so knock yourself out and eat up. <u>Anytime, and at any meal.</u> Even late night, vegetables will be our mainstay to curb hunger. Some diets may say that certain vegetables can lead to excess calories or fat retention, but to me that is a needless worry. No one gets fat by eating too many vegetables. That is an oxymoron. So for our purposes, we will eat them whenever we want!

FOOD CHART

Food	Category	Calories	Protein	Carbs
Beans, Black Beans	Carbohydrates	150	8	30
Bread, 9 or 12 Grain Bread	Carbohydrates	80	3	15
Bread, Rye Bread	Carbohydrates	90	3	15
Bread, Sourdough Bread	Carbohydrates	70	3	15
Bread, Whole Wheat Bread	Carbohydrates	70	3	13
Bread, Whole Wheat Pita	Carbohydrates	170	5	40
Fruit, Apple or Orange	Carbohydrates	100	0	30
Fruit, Apricots (3)	Carbohydrate	50	0	12
Fruit, Avocado (1/4)	Carbohydrates	80	0	4
Fruit, Banana	Carbohydrate	120	0	35
Fruit, Grapes (1 cup)	Carbohydrates	115	0	30
Fruit, Melon	Carbohydrates	135	0	30
Fruit, Nectarine	Carbohydrates	65	0	20
Fruit, Peach	Carbohydrates	75	0	20
Fruit, Pear	Carbohydrates	115	0	30
Fruit, Plum	Carbohydrates	30	0	7
Fruit, Raspberries (1 cup)	Carbohydrates	70	0	15
Fruit, Strawberries (1 cup)	Carbohydrates	50	0	11
Fruit, Watermelon	Carbohydrates	50	1	11
Grain, Barley	Carbohydrates	170	3	35
Oatmeal, Old Fashioned Oatmeal	Carbohydrates	150	5	30
Pasta, wheat	Carbohydrates	200	7	40
Potato, Baked Potato	Carbohydrates	220	5	50
Potato, Sweet Potato	Carbohydrates	150	5	45
Potato, Yam	Carbohydrates	150	5	45
Rice, Steamed Brown Rice	Carbohydrates	215	5	45
Rice, Steamed Wild Rice	Carbohydrates	170	5	35
Salsa (2 tbsp)	Carbohydrates	10	0	2
Wheat Germ	Carbohydrates	50	5	6

Note: Please, please, please do not fall victim to the backwards thinking of eating carbohydrates causes getting fat. What causes fat gain is the overindulgence of carbohydrates (and other foods), not the moderate intake of your body's preferred fuel. Remember, our carbohydrate intake is actually going to help us burn fat through the UP - DOWN plan! Just make sure the carbs you are choosing are on the guide. Be mindful of a portion.

FOOD CHART

Food	Category	Calories	Protein	Carbs
Flaxseeds or Flaxseed Oil (3 Tbsp)	Miscellaneous	180	9	12
Fudgsicle, no sugar added	Miscellaneous	45	-	9
Jell-O pudding, sugar free / fat free (made with fat free or skim milk)	Miscellaneous	80	-	8
Milk, fat free (1 cup)	Miscellaneous	80	9	12
Nuts, Almonds (1oz.)	Miscellaneous	165	6	6
Nuts, Peanuts (1oz. Dry roasted- no salt)	Miscellaneous	170	8	5
Nuts, Walnuts (1oz.) `	Miscellaneous	195	5	5
Olive Oil (1Tbsp.)	Miscellaneous	120	0	0
Yogurt, fat free (1 cup)	Miscellaneous	120	8	21

Note on nuts: Nuts pack a huge caloric punch so be careful. However I will never say to someone dieting that they have to deprive themselves of nuts. The nuts on the food guide provide great sources of heart healthy good fats, and also can satiate the appetite. Yet we have to remember serving size and make sure 1 ounce stays 1 ounce.

Note on fruit: I allow many different kinds of fruit on this plan, but I do shun fruit juice. So, instead of drinking orange juice, instead eat a fresh orange. Certain diets hate on fruit as well, and say that it will make us fat. Let us use our common sense here for a minute. Fruit in moderation makes us fat? This just is not true, as long as you are sticking to one piece of fruit and or 1 cup, if the guide says so. We need the nutrients and vitamins in our diets! Please don't be fooled into thinking fresh fruit is bad.

Note about serving size: Serving size has been spoken about earlier, however as a quick reminder, use the label on the food or a clenched fist for one serving of protein, carbs, and vegetables. For certain foods I have put the serving size next to it either in ounces, cups or tablespoons. You need to really stick to the serving size with these foods because over indulgence will lead to fat retention. Nuts for instance are very dense with calories, so make sure 1 ounce stays 1 ounce.

Chapter 5

Hotbody Lifting Program: The Equipment
Getting Comfortable With Gyms

True success is overcoming the fear of being unsuccessful. – Paul Seeney

It's More and Less Than You Think

Before I begin, I want to say that this program is perfect for both males and females, and has in fact worked for both! So any girls or guys out there who think it can't work or feel they don't know enough about gyms and fitness to do this need not be worried. Together we are going to change your body in only 8 to 10 weeks!

OK, so in this section we are tackling another one of the major roadblocks to getting in shape in college . . . the ability to navigate through the gym. I remember when I was in high school, I thought I knew everything there was to know about the gym. I knew what a bench was, and I knew what a curl bar was . . . 'nough said, right? I mean, aren't those the only two muscles that a guy needs? (Chest and biceps.) Hey, throw in a little abs and I might as well be Brad Pitt from "Fight Club" (or Demi Moore for the ladies).

I took the same routine with me to college. (Only now there were girls in the weight room, which definitely affected my approach.) I lifted on and off for my first two, two and half years. Let me tell you exactly what my program consisted of. I would go to the gym at about 10 at night and automatically find myself seated on the free weight bench. I'd do bout 5 sets with shit form and no idea of the amount of weight. As a guy, my whole goal was to be able to "throw up" (lift) two wheels (two 45 pound plates) on each side, a total of 225 pounds. (This is a common "guy goal.")

After my battle with the bench, (which never led to me being able to lift the two 45's . . . only when I changed my diet and exercise program did I achieve this and more), it was on to something called biceps curls. Here is the quick overview. I had a bar that looked like someone bent it a couple times (also known as the cambered bar). I would put too much weight on, and then use my back and legs to lift it, all the while thinking, "Damn right, I look good." During this show that I was putting on, I would also be checking to see which females would be looking my way. Boy, I was one smart guy. Girls really love a dude who looks like an ass in the gym, let me tell ya. Let alone one who is always looking to see if they are looking back at him.

Well, mistakes are meant to happen, no use living in the past. After 5 sets of this, I was just about done with lifting, and it was time to leave the gym and then return tomorrow night at the same time and do the exact same routine. (And I wondered why this wasn't working.) Hey hold on a second here . . . you know what? No one is born with a "get fit" gene. (see glossary) The gene that lets them know from birth exactly how to lift with perfect form, and what each piece of equipment is. That's right - I wasn't born with it and neither were you. We all have to learn, and this book is your tool to learn with. I promise you that after reading this book, you will know exactly what piece of equipment you need to work a certain body part upon entering every gym – and how to use it. That is why I have the pictures, because we are not born knowing this shit! Raise your hand if you know what a cambered bar or a leg extension machine is? Exactly, but you will.

The Equipment

I worked out in two gyms during my college tenure – one was the campus gym (ooh, fond memories . . .) and the other was the local Powerhouse Gym. (Now, I loved this place, but that is not to say your gym at school won't rival it. I loved it because the people that went there were into fitness and knew their stuff. I was first exposed to lifting from watching these guys do proper exercise techniques.)

As a certified trainer, I've learned that lifting technique and regimens can vary – and can be relatively simple, and still get the results you are after. You will find the **HotBody.101 Program** keeps it simple and relatively easy to do. Here is one thing I am sure of. I know that this program will work for you if you are consistent in your diet and exercise.

I am going to explain (and show you via photos) each piece of equipment in the gym that you need to be familiar with in order to complete the program.

Dumbbells

Dumbbells are by far my favorite piece of equipment in the gym. They are easily the most versatile and can and will be used for pressing, raising, curling, and extending.

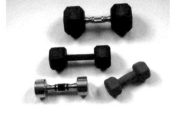

Flat Bench and or Incline Bench

This can come as an incline version or flat version, it will fold into whichever position. Or another type of bench is the one that is simply a bench. It is rectangular and can not be made into an incline version.

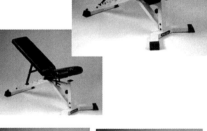

Pulldown Machine

This machine is called a pulldown machine for one reason. You pull the weight down. The fun thing about this is that you can switch the grip and bars you use to pull with. We will switch the bars within the program from wide grip bar, to short straight bar, to a V-bar. (These two pictures show a wide grip bar and a V-bar.)

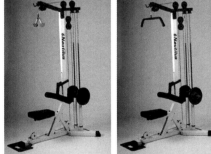

Leg Extension Machine

This machine is the one where you extend your legs. It might be set on a slight incline, which is fine.

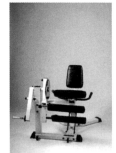

Leg Curl Machine
Yup, this one you curl your legs. This machine might be offered lying on your stomach, or standing up, that is fine too.

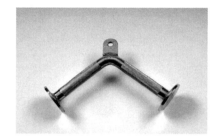

V-bar
Common sense tells us this bar looks just like the letter V. You see, this program is user friendly!

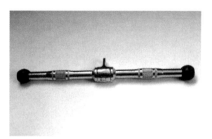

Straight bar (short)
Bet you already know that this bar is short and straight.

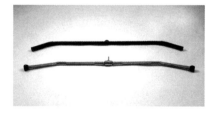

Wide grip bar
This bar is long and has angled ends, as you can see by the picture.

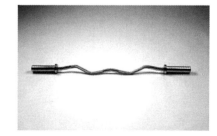

Cambered Bar (Bent)
This is the bar that looks bent at the ends.

Want To Work Out At Home?

If you want to invest between $300 and $500, you can set up a "home gym" situation in your apartment or home that will give you the benefits of this work out program. I would recommend a sturdy adjustable bench (approximately $225) and the Personal Powerblock Set (approximately $220) or a basic dumbbell set (approximately $50). (An excellent place to do this would be Leisure Fitness, they provide excellent equipment at reasonable prices.) You also might have a Bowflex or other complete machine. That is great! This program can work at home with just the addition of some dumbbells! Please take advantage of contacting me by e-mail if you have any questions at all about the exercises or anything at all! I will do my best to respond in a timely manner.

Next Up . . .

Learn how to USE the equipment to get your *HotBody*!

Chapter 6

HotBody Lifting Program:
The Exercises

They always say time changes things, but you actually have to change them yourself.
– Andy Warhol

Let's Get Started!
Each exercise is described in text and illustrated in photos. This chapter shows you how to do each exercise. Be sure to try each exercise FIRST without the weights, to get a feel for the motion. Start with light weight. Once you are familiar with the exercises, you will be ready to set up your workout schedule and get going!

MENU OF EXERCISES
Here are all the approved exercises you will do for each body part. The program you select (10-week or 8-week) will guide you in the exercises you will do.

> **To get a starting weight -**
> Pick a weight that you can comfortably do 12 reps with (before fatigue) but not so light that you are easily doing 14-15 reps.

NOTE: *All exercises that are performed in the pictures by one hand or on one side are also done on the opposite side or with the opposite hand as well. Therefore, if it says 12 reps for one arm dumbbell row, that means 12 reps each side would equal one set. Also, you might notice our female model Courtney's feet not totally on the floor in a few of the pictures with the bench and or incline bench. This is fine, she felt most comfortable this way and I recommend that you do what feels most comfortable to you as well. This program is not supposed to cause great pain. Instead, you should really feel the muscle working while being comfortable in your form. One last thing, the exercise toes out calf raises is the only one not pictured. It is however exactly how it sounds. You stand on the floor with your toes angled so your feet look like a V in front of you. You simply rise up and down on your toes.*

Chest
Dumbbell flat bench press
Dumbbell incline bench press
Flyes
Push ups

Back
Wide grip pulldowns
Narrow grip pulldowns
Reverse grip pulldowns
One arm dumbbell rows

Hamstrings Quads
Dumbbell squat
Dumbbell lunges
Leg extensions
Leg curls

Shoulders
Upright rows
Lateral raise (to the side)
Front raises
Dumbbell rear shoulder raises (seated)
Shoulder press

Traps
Dumbbell shrugs (optional for girls)

Calves
Regular weighted calf raises
Incline (on a step) toe raises
Toes out calf raises

Biceps
*Dumbbell incline bench rotating biceps
   curl*
Hammer curls
*Cambered bar (crooked bar) standing
   curls*

Triceps
*Overhead dumbbell extensions V-bar
   pushdowns*
Reverse grip straight bar extensions

Abs
Crunch
Leg up

Dumbbell flat bench press [Chest]

Yup, you guessed it you will need a flat bench to do this exercise. Any college gym will have one.

- o   Lie on your back on a bench so that your upper and mid back are flush.
- o   Hold a dumbbell in each hand.
- o   Move the dumbbells to a point just above your shoulders. Keep your elbows pointing away and the palm of your hand facing a point just above feet level.
- o   Begin to move the weights up in an arc like motion so that at the top they rest just above your upper chest. Do not lockout your arms, meaning always keep a slight bend in your elbows so as to relieve stress on your joints.
- o   Slowly bring the weight back to a starting position and thus you have completed one rep! Good job!

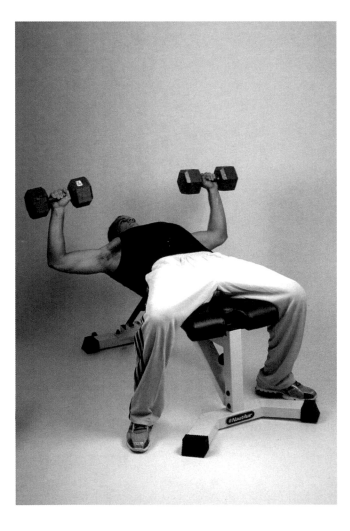
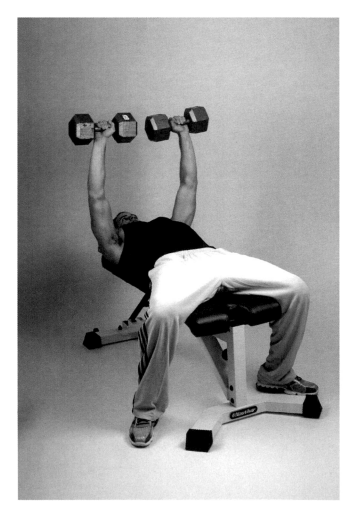

Dumbbell incline bench press [Chest]

- o Lie back on an incline bench set at approximately 130 degrees. Hold a dumbbell in each hand so they are chest level and your arms are at 90 degrees.

- o Move the dumbbells up in an arcing motion so that they are about 4 inches from being together when your arms are extended. Make sure the dumbbells are centered over your upper chest to chin area.

- o Slowly lower them back into place to complete the rep.

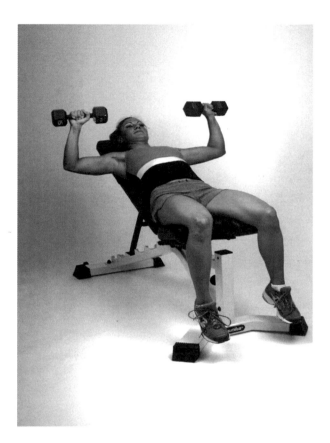

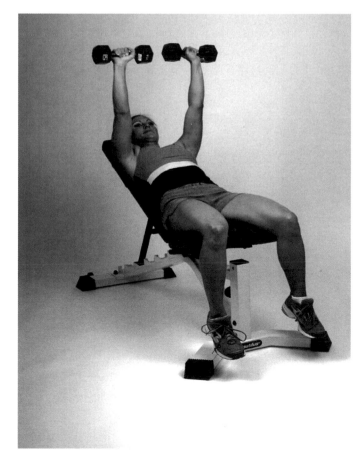

Dumbbell flyes [Chest]

I read somewhere that you should think of it as hugging a tree. Well for three years that is what I have been picturing, and you want to know what? That is exactly the motion.

- o Begin lying back on an incline bench. Bring the weight up like you were performing a bench press, but instead rotate your grip so your palms face each other.
- o Begin the motion of hugging a tree. The movement should be an arc ending with the weights about 4 inches apart.

Always keep a slight bend in your motion and upon reaching the top, lower slowly back down to the original position.

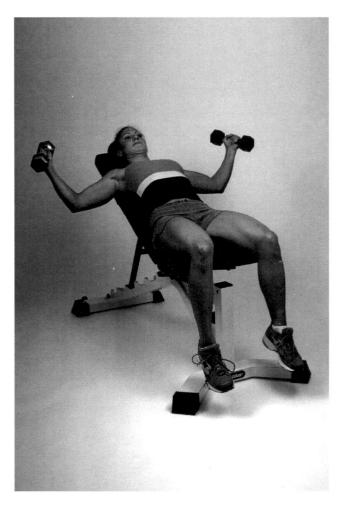

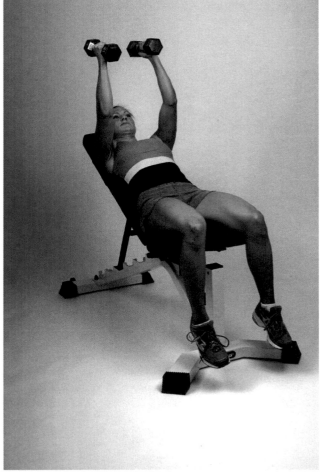

Push Ups [Chest]

- o   Assume a push up position, feet about 2 inches apart and hands about an inch past shoulder width.

- o   Slowly lower yourself until your chest is an inch above the ground.

- o   Slowly raise yourself back up to the starting position.

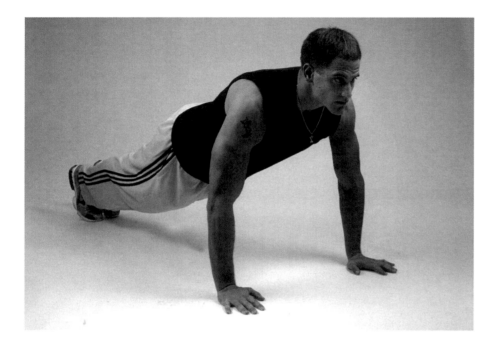

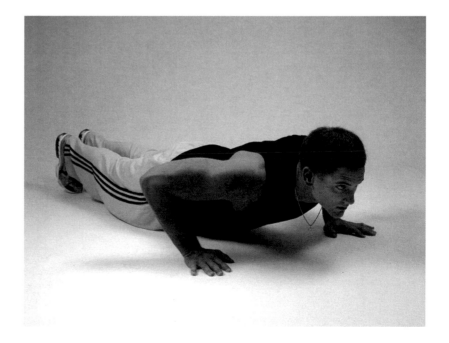

Wide grip pulldowns [Back]

- o Locate a pulldown machine and sit in it.

- o Using a Wide grip bar (it is bent at the ends), take a grip right where the bend occurs.

- o Keep your back straight during the exercise with as little lean as you can allow.

- o Make sure that your knees are fitting comfortably tight underneath the kneepads.

- o Begin by pulling the bar down to the top of your chest, pause a second and then slowly let the weight return to the beginning position.

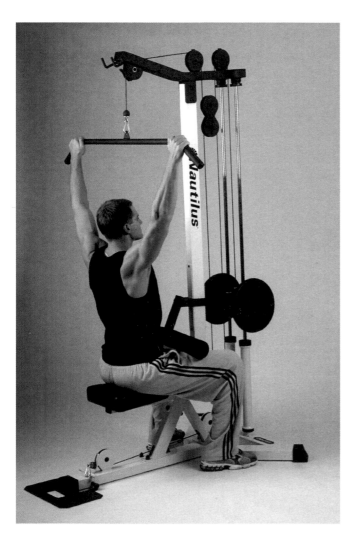

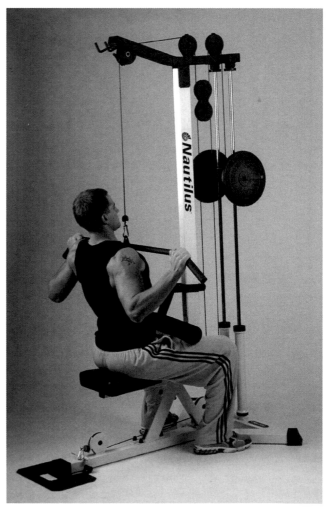

Narrow grip pulldowns [Back]

o   Same as wide grip just with a narrow grip.

o   Your hands should be about 6 inches apart.

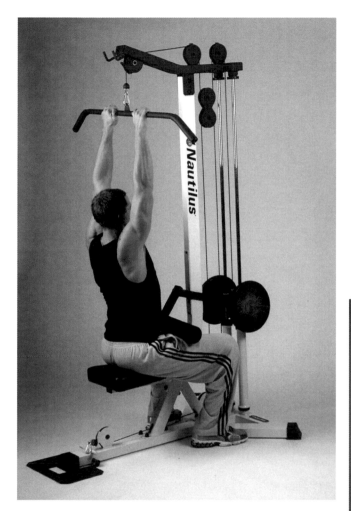

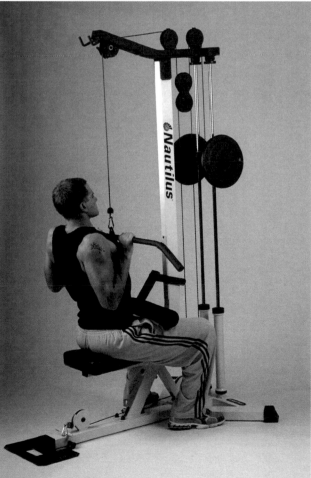

Reverse grip pulldowns [Back]

- o   Same motion as all of the other pulldowns, just with your grip reversed (palms facing you).
- o   Keep your hands about 6 inches apart.

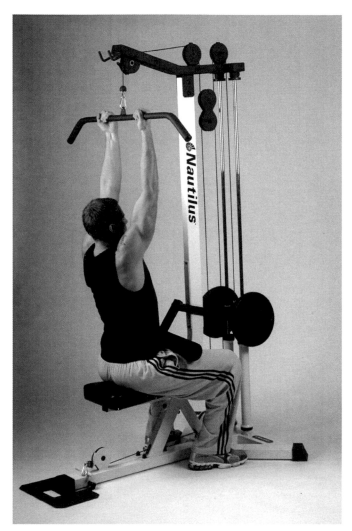

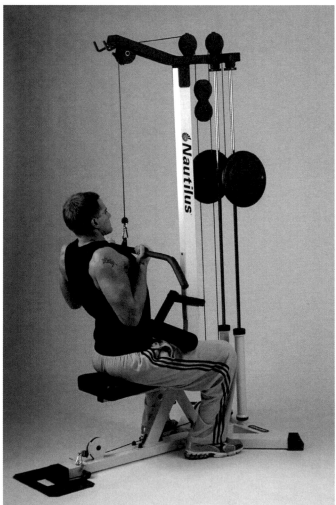

One arm dumbbell rows [Back]

(Quick tip, always keep your head up! Also keep your back straight and flat.)

- o Find yourself a bench a dumbbell.
- o We will start right arm first, so you need to put your left knee up on the bench and have your right leg planted to the floor bend over and put your left hand on the bench and let the dumbbell hang from your right hand.
- o Keep your eyes and head forward and raise the weight until it is touching your chest.
- o Slowly lower it back into starting position. (after completing the number of reps for one side, switch to the other and complete the same number of reps)

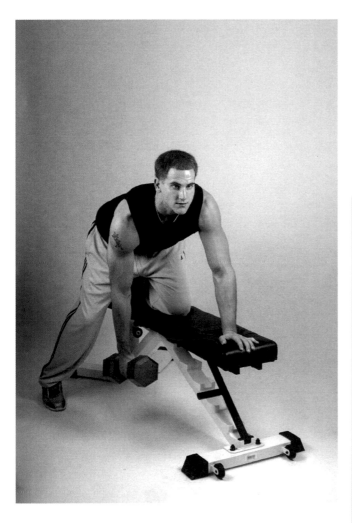

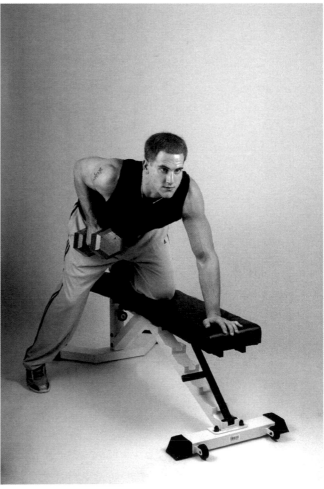

Dumbbell squats [Legs]

- o With two dumbbells in both hands, assume a standing position with your feet about a foot apart.

- o With your head up and eyes looking straight ahead, begin to bend down at your knees with your back staying straight.

- o When your thighs are parallel to the floor, begin to raise back up to the starting position.

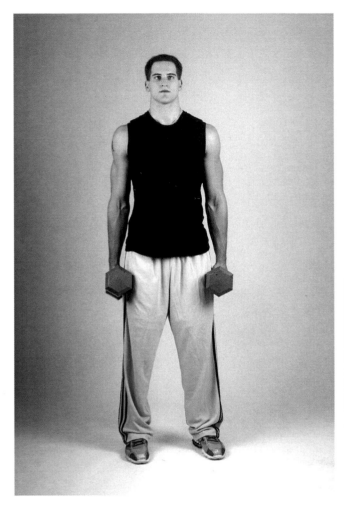

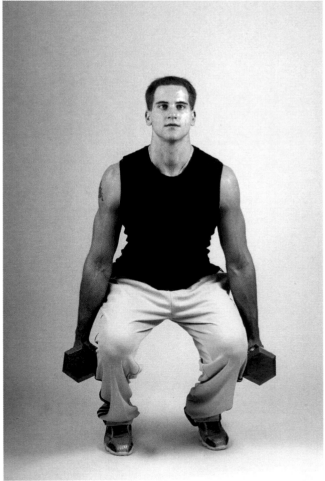

Dumbbell lunges [Legs]

(So you guys out there think these look funny? Try them and then tell me what you think. I'll tell you right now, they are not easy to do, and will really give your legs a thrashing.)

- Grab a dumbbell for each hand and stand in an erect position. (Very funny . . . haha erect . . . ok back to the exercise . . .)

- Keep your gaze forward and your chin level with the floor. Make sure your back is not tilted, try to be as straight as possible.

- Step forward and bend at the knee until your other knee is just about at the floor . . . (4 inches or so above it)

- Push up with that leg and return to the starting position.

- Do the same for the opposite leg. (Keep your toes and foot in line. Basically try not to point them out or in.)

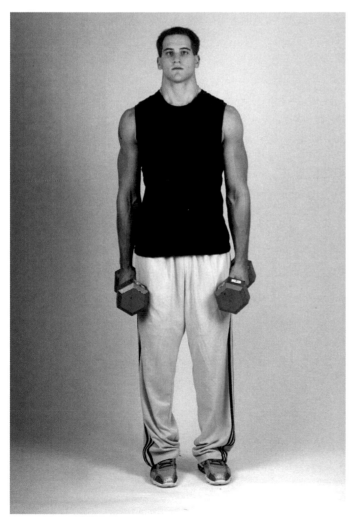
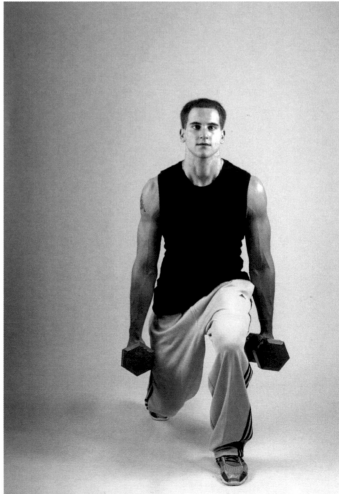

Leg extension [Legs]

This machine is the one where you extend your legs. It might be set on a slight incline – that is fine.

- o   Sit down and place your ankles behind the pad.
- o   Rest it on your lower shins.
- o   Straighten your legs. As you do so the weight will rise.
- o   Go for a good extension of almost parallel and then return slowly to the beginning position.

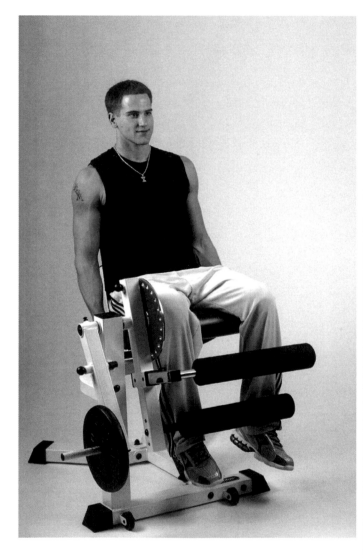
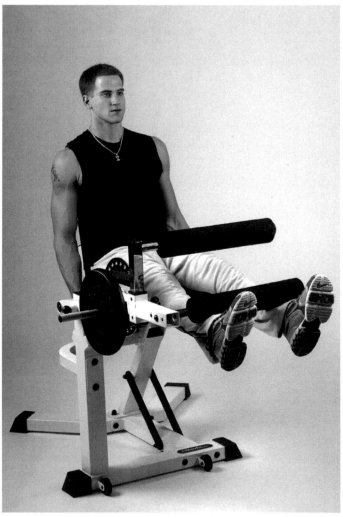

Leg curls [Legs]

Yup, this one you curl your legs. This machine might be offered lying on your stomach, or standing up—either way is fine.

- Either lie down or sit down, or stand with your ankles touching the pads.
- Curl up your legs until they almost touch your butt.
- Pause a second and then slowly lower the pad/weight to its starting position.

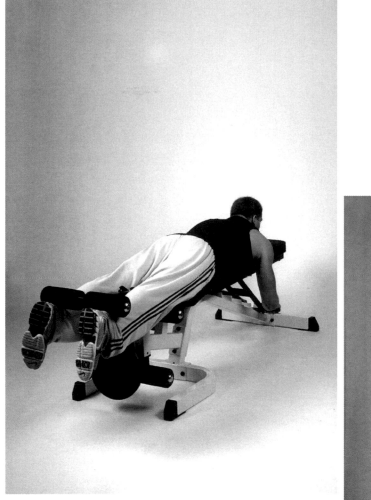

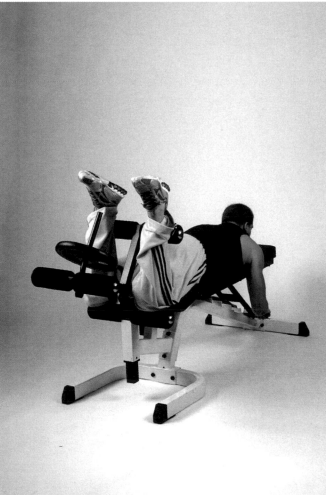

Upright rows (with a cambered bar...the bent one) [Shoulders]

o Begin by standing with your feet about ten inches apart and holding a cambered bar at the bent angles with an overhand grip with both hands (start with a very slight bend in the elbows to avoid total lockout).

o Raise the bar up and toward your chin, this process will cause your elbows to flare out to the sides.

When the weight is a couple inches below the chin, begin to lower it back to the starting position.

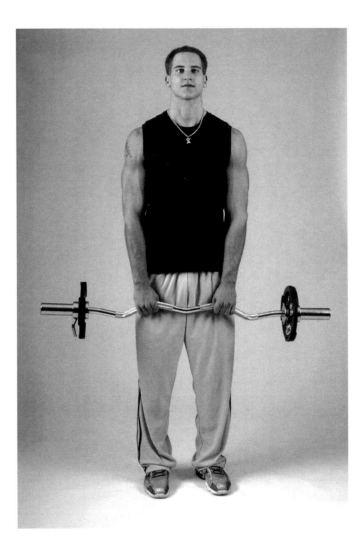

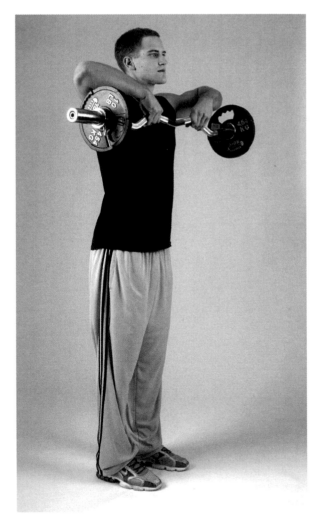

Dumbbell front raises [Shoulders]

This is as simple as it sounds. Front raises are as follows.

- o   Grasp two dumbbells in your hands palms facing in. You are simply raising one in front of you until it reaches eye level.

- o   Upon reaching eye level you will then lower it in a controlled manner.

- o   When the dumbbell has returned to the starting position you will raise the other one in the same fashion.

- o   Count one rep with both hands as one total rep. (So that means both hands have to have lifted the weight once each to count for one total rep. I like to take the cadence of one, one . . . two, two)

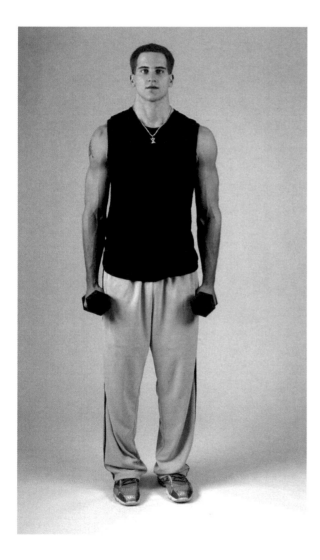

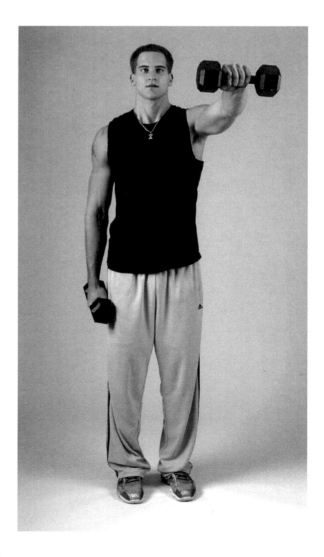

Dumbbell lateral raise - side [Shoulders]

- o Just like front raises, except you are lifting the weight out to your sides.

- o Once you reach what I like to call the T position you will slowly lower the weights. (T position is one where your arms are out to the side so your body resembles a T.)

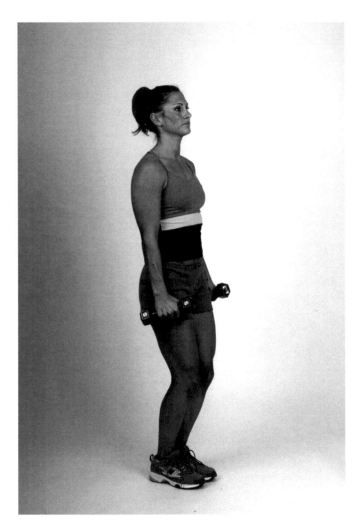

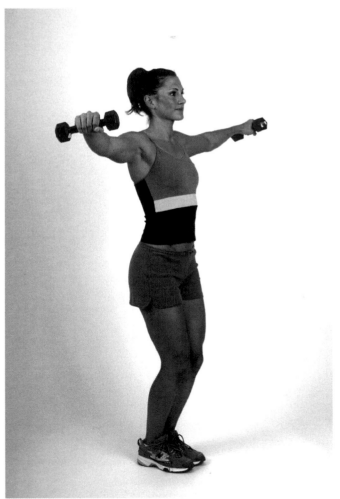

Dumbbell rear shoulder raise - (seated) [Shoulders]

(This exercise is a favorite of mine, but can often be performed wrong. Many people in the gym will look at you like "what the hell is he/she doing"? - but those who have some knowledge will know you are doing the exercise right.)

- o Start by sitting on the end of a bench with your feet flat in front of you and your chest nearly touching your knees.

- o Your eyes are looking ahead of you, which allows your head to be up.

- o You will lift both weights out to the side much like a side lateral raise, but the angle at which you are working will mainly isolate the real deltoid.

- o Once you are in your quasi T position (or your "I'm a flying squirrel" position, cause this is what you will look like) you will lower the weights slowly back down.

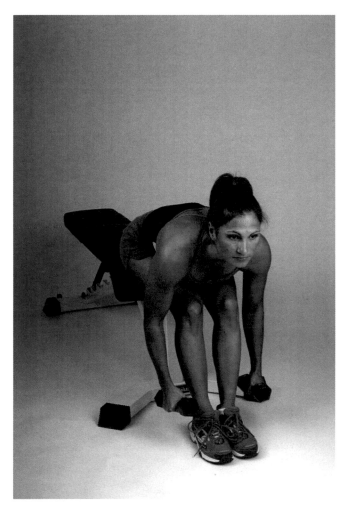

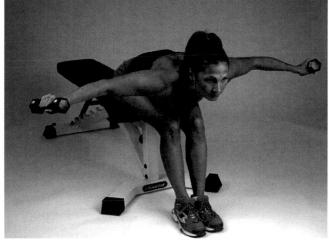

Dumbbell shoulder press (seated) [Shoulders]

o   Find an Incline bench and position it in an "L".

o   Sit down back against the bench.

o   Bring both dumbbells over you head so you look like T position but your arms are bent 90 degrees.

o   Keep your palms facing forward and your elbows pointing away.

o   Move the dumbbells in an arcing manner so they come close to touching above your head, but don't quite get there, all the while extend your arms so they are almost straight up and down.

o   Bring the weight back down slowly to the starting position and make sure all the while your gaze is ahead of you, not up towards the dumbbells.

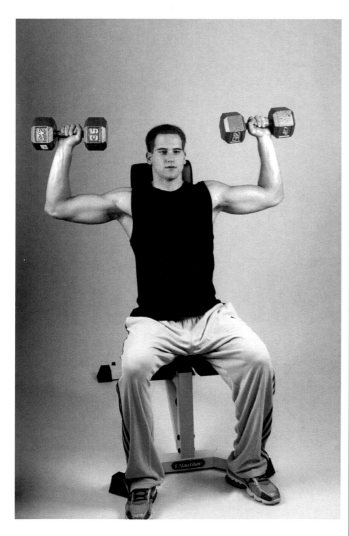
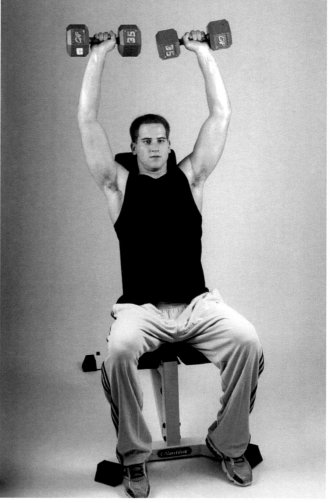

Dumbbell shrugs [Traps]

NOTE: Optional for girls (most girls I know don't want to have huge traps, on the other hand many guys do. In fact our fitness model, Courtney, does not do these and as you can see, she still looks great!)

- o Grab two dumbbells in both hands and take a stance that allows your knees to have a slight bend.

- o Allow both dumbbells to hang down by your sides in a hammer grip.

- o Slowly raise your shoulders so that you try to touch your shoulders to your ears. (This is of course impossible but that is the motion you are going for.)

DO NOT rotate your shoulders back or forward in any motion. Just plain up and down. Any rotation will put undue stress on the joints.

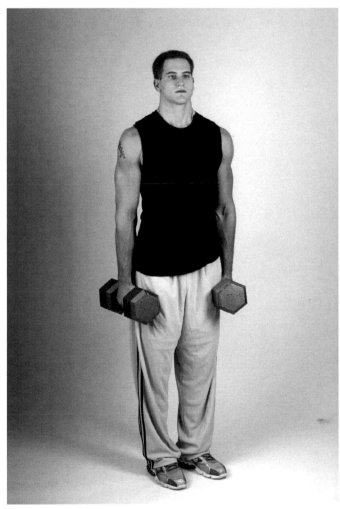
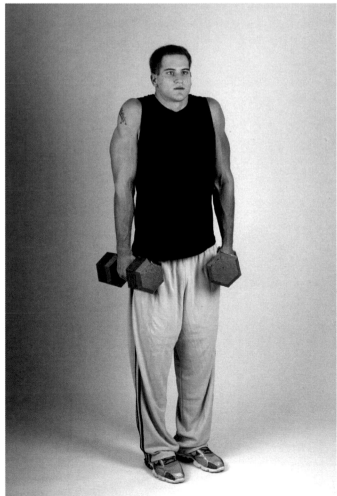

Regular weighted calf raises [calves]

- o   Begin by grabbing a weight for both hands and assume a standing position with your view straight ahead.

- o   Begin by raising up on your toes and try to achieve the greatest stretch you feel possible.

- o   Hold for a second and then slowly lower down until your heels touch the floor.

- o   At this point you will begin the exercise again for the allotted number of Reps.

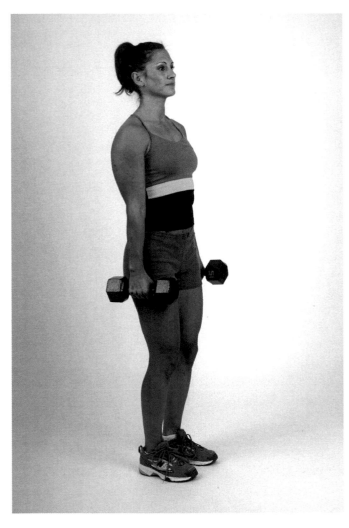

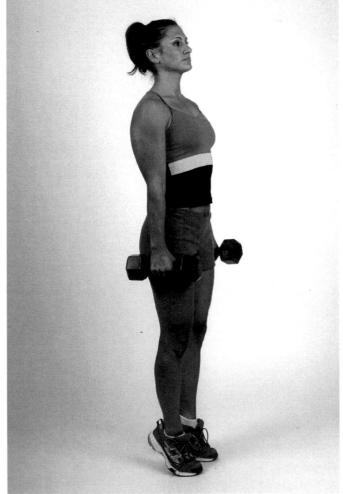

Incline (on your biggest book or a step) toe raises [calves]

- o Find your biggest book and put it down on the floor (can also do this exercise using the edge of a step, if you've already lost you biology 101 book).
- o Also find something that you can balance on like a stool or chair.
- o Stand on the end of the book with your toes about two inches onto the end of the book.
- o Lower your heels all the way down to right above the ground.
- o Raise up using your toes and calf muscles until you feel the greatest stretch.
- o Slowly lower your body down to the original start position.

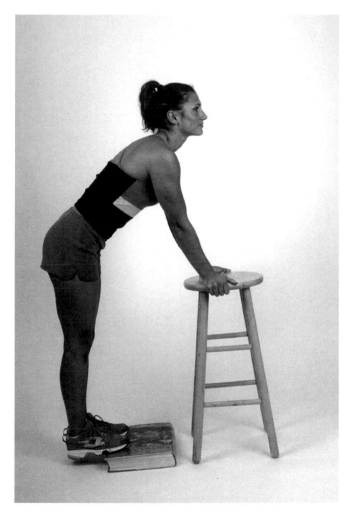
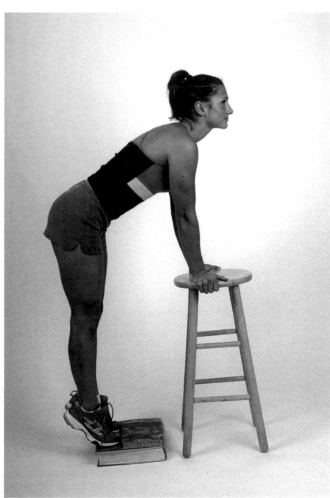

Dumbbell incline bench rotating bicep curl [Biceps]

Woohoo big words, but really a simple movement . . . You'll see!

- o Sit back on an incline bench set at about 45 degrees.

- o Keep your head up and your sight facing forward.

- o Keep the two dumbbells hanging at your side palms facing your side.

- o Slowly begin to curl them up.

- o At the midpoint of the curl you are to begin to supinate (rotate your wrist) so that at the end of the motion your palms will face the ceiling.

- o This is a little tricky to start with, but once you get the hang of it, it really becomes not only easy, but an enjoyable exercise, since you will be "peaking your biceps" each time you curl. That means you will see your arms making a muscle. Your arms should be at a 30-degree angle at the top of the curl, and then you will slowly lower the weight back into the starting position.

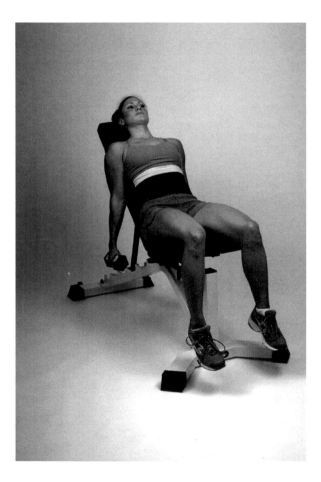

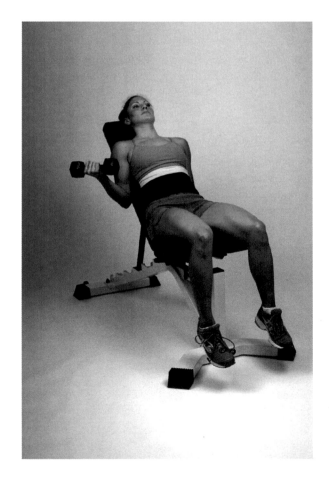

Dumbbell hammer curls [Biceps]

- o Basically you are holding the weight like you would a hammer. There is no rotation in this exercise.

- o Stand with your feet at about shoulder width distance and a slight bend in your knees.

- o Grasp the two dumbbells in a hammer grip. (Palms facing in) Raise each dumbbell separately using the one-one, two-two cadence. The weight will be raised straight up to a 30-degree angle of your arms. Slowly return the weight to its original starting position. There is no movement of the wrist through out this motion, your wrist stays stationary.

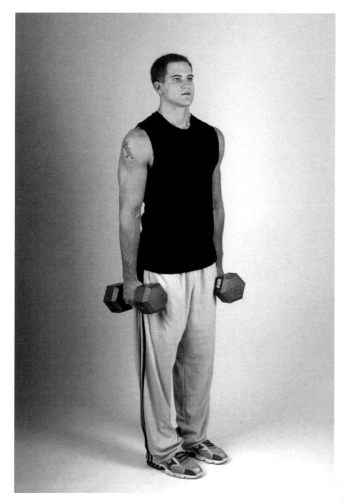

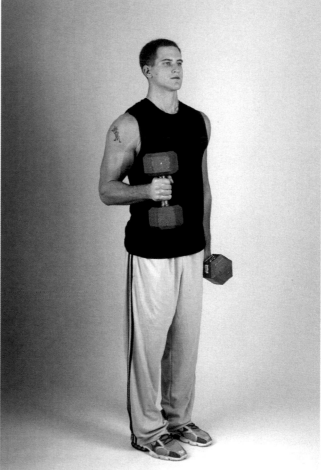

Cambered bar (crooked bar) standing curls [Biceps]

- o Begin by standing with your feet about ten inches apart and holding a cambered bar at the bent angles with an underhand grip with both hands (start with a very slight bend in the elbows to avoid total lockout).

- o Begin to raise (curl) the weight up.

- o When you have achieved a 15 to 20 degree angle, pause and then slowly lower the weight back to the original starting position.

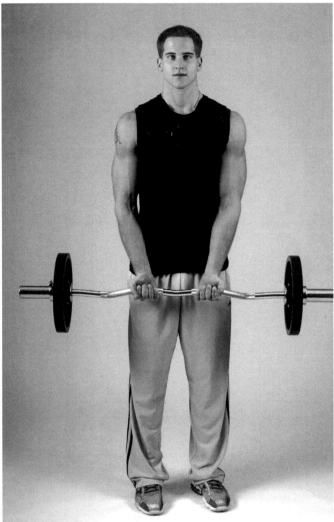
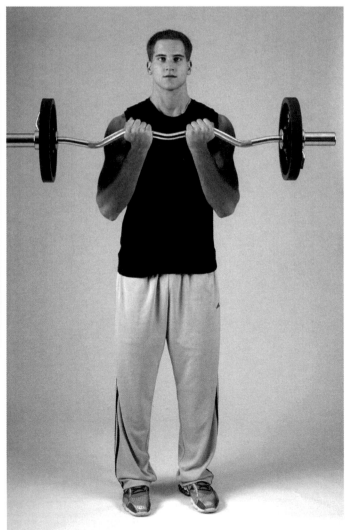

Overhead dumbbell extension [Triceps]

Be careful to use a weight that you can definitely control!

- o   Find a dumbbell that feels comfortable to hold as seen in the pictures.
- o   Find an incline bench (set to a position that looks like an "L") and sit down with your back pressed against the bench.
- o   Grab one end of the dumbbell with both hands and raise it over your head in an outstretched position.
- o   Slowly lower it behind your head until you reach a 90-degree angle with your arms.
- o   Raise the weight to its original position and that is one rep.

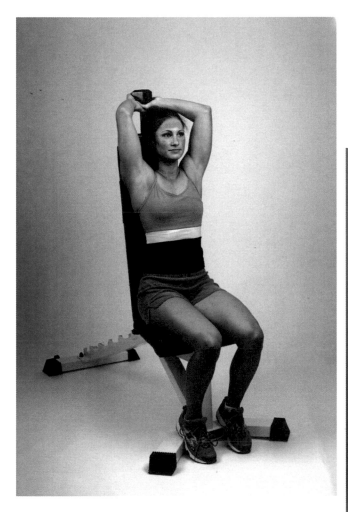
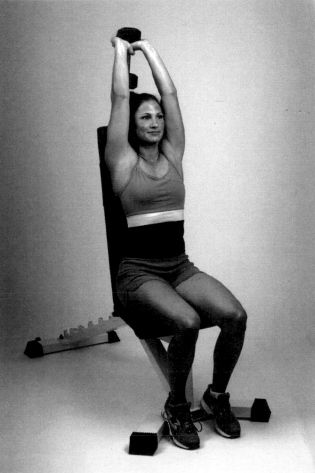

V-bar tricep pushdown [Triceps]

- o Grab a V-bar and attach it to the high cable machine.

- o The starting point for this exercise will be with your arms at 90 degrees.

- o Your body will be straight with a little bend in your knees.

- o With your arms in the starting position, push the weight down so that your arms are almost straight with a slight bend at the elbows.

- o Try to keep your elbows touching your sides the whole time. (Keep them in basically.)

- o Return the weight to the 90-degree position and that is one rep.

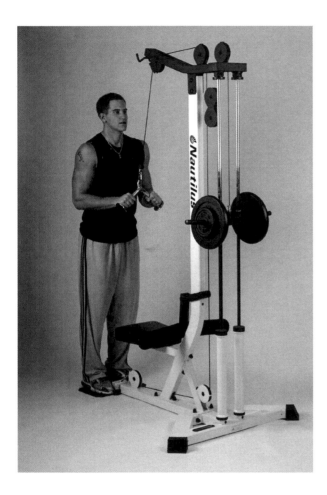

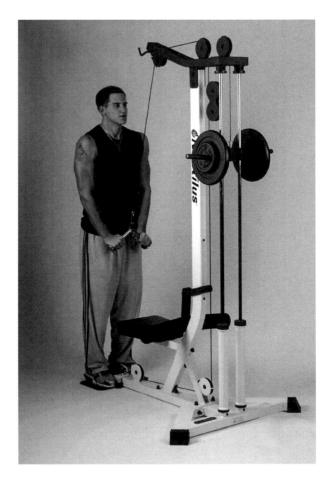

Reverse grip straight bar extension [Triceps]

Same deal as regular pushdowns, with a different bar and different grip.

- o Grab a straight pushdown bar and use a reverse grip. (Just a heads up – a reverse grip is palms facing you.)
- o The movement, however, mimics the regular pushdown.

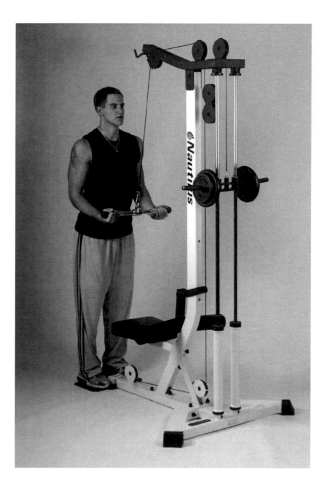

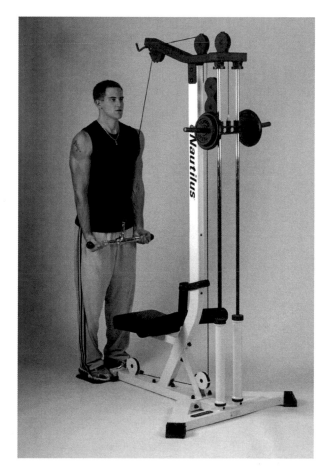

Michael S. Kamins

Crunch [Abs]

- o Start on the floor, lying down with your knees drawn up.

- o Place your hands either behind your head or across your chest and begin to lift up using your abdominals.

- o This range of motion is very short, so you should only be lifting your shoulders off the ground about 5 inches.

- o Once you have held this position for a good second lower back down.

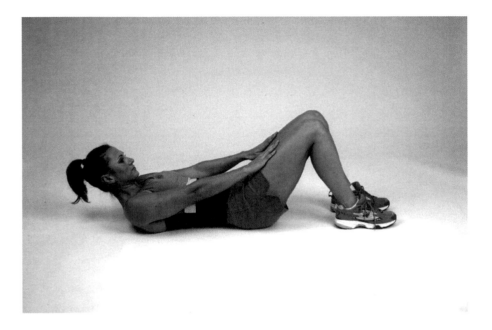

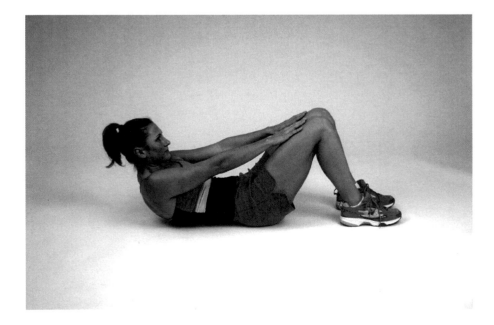

Leg Up [Abs]

- o Begin by lying flat on the floor with your legs straight out and touching, and your hands slightly under your butt.

- o Slowly raise your legs up until they are a little past 90 degrees and your hips have just begun to leave the floor.

- o Pause and return to starting position.

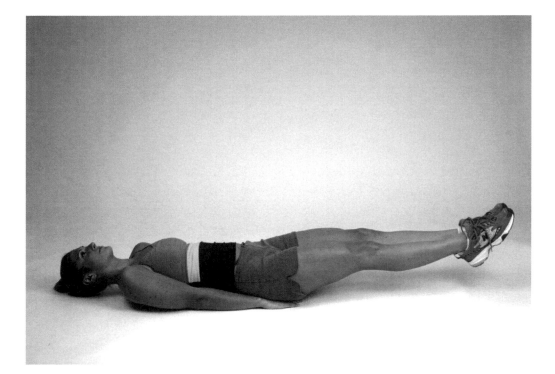

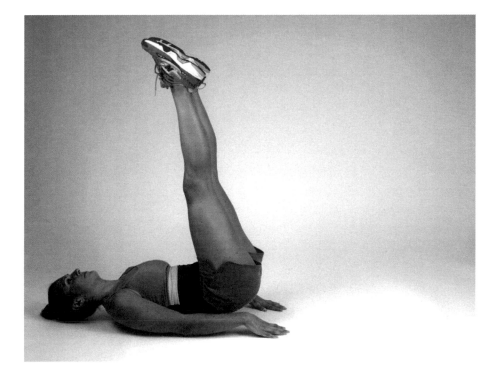

Chapter 7

HotBody Lifting Program:
The Workout

*Always bear in mind that your own resolution to succeed is more important
than any one thing.*
—Abraham Lincoln

First of all, know this. Lifting weights will burn fat and increase metabolism. (Hear that ladies and gents? Cardio is great but won't do it all. You have to lift to get the *HotBody* look.) OK, like I said earlier, you can choose to lift either three or ve days a week. Below is the breakdown of muscle groups for each of the plans.

FIVE DAY PLAN (results in 8 weeks)

I lift Monday through Friday, but you can use any five days in a 7-day week. I picked this so I could have the weekends free of lifting, and only have to worry about cardio . . . you can choose whatever five days work best for your schedule. Below are the days of the week and corresponding muscle groups you will work.

Monday	Chest and Calves
Tuesday–	Back and Abs
Wednesday	Hamstrings and Quadriceps . . .
	(a.k.a. legs, minus the calves)
Thursday	Shoulders, Traps and Calves
Friday	Arms and Abs baby . . . oh yea!
	(Friday should be a fun day anyway-right?)

THREE DAY PLAN (results in 10 weeks)

Ok, so you're opting for the ten week plan. That's fine, it will work just as well! You may have more time to reach your goal, or you simply may rather lift only three days a week. Whatever the reason, the point is that ten weeks from now you are going to be sporting your HotBody!

The lifting phase is broken down into three days a week. Cardio will still be every other day. Now cardio and lifting might be on the same day, or might not, it just depends on how you decide to set up your schedule. I will use Monday, Wednesday, and Friday as lifting days, and cardio would then be Sunday, Tuesday, Thursday, and Saturday. Everyone is different so the time of day you choose to do these is up to you! Hell, I usually had late classes in college, mostly after 12, others had the 8 in the morning classes, you just have to decide what days and times are best for you. So, without further ado....

Monday	Chest, Back, Calves, and Abs
Wednesday	Shoulders, Traps, Hamstrings, Abs
Friday	Arms, Quads, Abs

TECHNIQUES AND REPETITIONS

We will be talking about repetitions and sets. Here's what they mean.

> **Repetition** – The act of moving the weight through the designed arc of motion and back again to the starting position. This would equal one rep.

> **Set** – A set is the performing of an exercise for a given number of reps. For example, if I do 12 reps of chest press as a warm up, that is *one set*.

We will always do a warm up set no matter what. Every time we switch exercise a warm up set will be done. This will allow for a warming of the muscle and gives you a chance to become accustomed to the exercise.

TWO STAGES FOR EACH PLAN

I have broken down the program into two stages. Either the first and last five weeks of the 10 week plan, or the first five and last three weeks of the 8 week plan. You will have two stages, regardless of whether you lift three or five times a week. Stage One is the "get acquainted" phase. Stage Two kicks everything into high gear. No matter which plan you choose, Stage One will last for the initial five weeks.

(Although my program lasts 8-10 weeks, I want you to know that it will be increasingly beneficial if you <u>continue</u> with it, or some sort of diet and exercise program. When continuing the plan past eight or ten weeks, rotate each stage by each week on the plan)

Stage One – Stage one is the getting acquainted phase. During these five weeks you will do the exercise as described below in technique and repetitions area.

- Between each set you will rest for 45 seconds to a minute and then begin your next set of the same exercise until it is complete.

- Upon completion you will go to the next exercise and perform the reps and sets in the same manner.

- Please keep your rest period to a minute at the most since our goal here is to burn as much fat as possible.

Stage Two – Stage two will begin the sixth week of your program. Stage two is where we are going to seriously kick ass and burn the fat. Here is the trick, it's called compound sets. You will notice that there is always an even number of exercises that we do. This is for a reason. Beginning in the sixth week we will group numbers 1 and 2 together, 3 and 4, 5 and 6, and 7 and 8. **(The one exception is on Wednesday of the 3-day plan, since the 9th exercise is optional. The exercise is shoulder shrugs, and if you choose to do them, just do them last.)**

Let's take chest and abs day as an example. Exercise one is incline dumbbell press, and exercise two is leg ups. We will be doing what is called a compound set with these exercises. It works like this.

- Complete your first set of the incline presses, and immediately go and do a set of leg ups.

- NO REST in between. The rest period comes after you have done one set with inclines and one set with leg ups. You will rest 45 seconds to one minute and then repeat until all 8 sets of exercise 1 and 2 are complete.

- Then we will move onto exercises 3 and 4, same deal.

- 5 and 6, you guessed it same deal. And finally 7 and 8 are done in the same manner.

Compound sets *(stage 2)* will give you a great pump and keep you active the whole lifting session. An added bonus is that your workouts will no doubt end quicker. So you'll have more time to go shopping for a swimsuit!

FIVE DAY WORKOUT

	Exercise	Sets*	Reps
Monday - Chest and Calves			
#1	Incline dumbbell chest press	4	12-10-10-8
#2	Standing calf raises (biggest text book or step)	4	30-25-20-15
#3	Flat bench dumbbell press	4	12-10-10-8
#4	Weighted calf raise	4	16-14-12-10
#5	Dumbbell Flyes	4	12-10-10-8
#6	Pushups (no warm up)	3	12 to 15
Tuesday - Back and Abs			
#1	Wide grip pull down	4	12-10-10-8
#2	One arm dumbbell row	4	12-10-10-8
#3	Leg Ups	4	12-10-10-8
#4	Crunch on the floor	4	30-25-20-15
#5	Narrow grip pull downs	4	12-10-10-8
#6	Reverse grip pull downs	4	12-10-10-8
Wednesday - Hamstrings and Quads			
#1	Dumbbell Squat	4	12-10-10-8
#2	Leg extension	4	12-10-10-8
#3	Dumbbell lunges	4	12-10-10-8
#4	Leg curl	4	12-10-10-8
Thursday - Shoulders, Calves and Traps			
#1	Dumbbell shoulder press	4	12-10-10-8
#2	Dumbbell rear shoulder raise	4	12-10-10-8
#3	Standing calf (biggest textbook or step)	4	30-25-20-15
#4	Dumbbell shoulder shrug	4	12-10-10-8
#5	Upright rows	4	12-10-10-8
#6	Weighted calf raise	4	16-14-12-10
#7	Dumbbell forward shoulder raise	4	12-10-10-8
#8	Toes out calves raises	4	20-18-16-14
Friday - Arms and Abs			
#1	Leg Ups	4	18-16-14-12
#2	Cambered bar (crooked bar) standing curls	4	12-10-10-8
#3	Seated overhead triceps extension	4	12-10-10-8
#4	Dumbbell incline bench rotating biceps curl	4	12-10-10-8
#5	V-Bar press downs	4	12-10-10-8
#6	Crunch on the floor (really try to feel the squeeze)	4	30-25-20-15
#7	Hammer Curls	4	12-10-10-8
#8	Reverse grip straight bar extensions	4	12-10-10-8

First set is always a warm up(except for push ups)

THREE DAY WORKOUT

	Exercise	Sets	Reps
Monday - Chest, Back, Calves, and Abs			
#1	Incline dumbbell chest press	4	12-10-10-8
#2	Flat bench dumbbell press	4	12-10-10-8
#3	Flyes	4	12-10-10-8
#4	Wide grip pull down	4	12-10-10-8
#5	One arm dumbbell row	4	12-10-10-8
#6	Leg ups	4	12-10-10-8
#7	Crunch on the floor	4	30-25-20-15
#8	Standing calf (biggest textbook or step)	4	16-14-12-10
Wednesday – Shoulders, Traps, Hamstrings, Abs			
#1	Dumbbell shoulder press	4	12-10-10-8
#2	Dumbbell rear shoulder raise	4	12-10-10-8
#3	Upright rows or side lateral raises (your choice)	4	12-10-10-8
#4	Dumbbell forward shoulder raise	4	12-10-10-8
#5	Crunch on the floor (really try to feel the squeeze)	4	30-25-20-15
#6	Leg curl	4	12-10-10-8
#7	Dumbbell lunges	4	12-10-10-8
#8	Leg Ups	4	18-16-14-12
#9	Shoulder shrug (optional)	4	12-10-10-8
Friday - Arms, Quads and Abs			
#1	Cambered bar (crooked bar) standing curls	4	12-10-10-8
#2	Seated overhead triceps extension	4	12-10-10-8
#3	Dumbbell incline bench rotating biceps curl	4	12-10-10-8
#4	V-Bar press downs	4	12-10-10-8
#5	Hammer Curls	4	12-10-10-8
#6	Reverse grip straight bar extensions	4	12-10-10-8
#7	Leg extension	4	12-10-10-8
#8	Dumbbell lunges	4	12-10-10-8
#9	Leg Ups	4	18-16-14-12
#10	Crunch on the floor (really try to feel the squeeze)	4	30-25-20-15

Chapter 8

HotBody Cardio: Three-Way Rotation

For success, try aspiration, inspiration, and perspiration. – Unattributed

I believe that the best way to burn fat is by doing cardio. There is no way around it! However, I don't necessarily believe in hours and hours of boring cardio in what doctors call the target heart rate zone. But, you <u>do</u> need to continuously rotate your cardio options. No option should be performed more than two days in a row. Here are the three options. (Remember from Chapter 2 - The Basics, that cardio needs to be done at least every other day.)

- *40 minutes of steady cardio at a moderate pace.* Moderate pace equals the ability to have a conversation while exercising although breathing is labored. (A normal jogging pace, not walking, jogging)

- *25-30 minutes based on intensity.* Warm up with 5 minutes at a moderate pace. Then proceed to increase resistance at every minute going to a preset maximum no higher than 4 above base level (that you will decide on based on comfort) either in resistance or incline for 18 minutes. Upon reaching the maximum, drop to original pace and repeat the increase every minute. For example, if your initial pace is 5, then switch every minute, 1 increment –like this -> 5, 6, 7, 8 – then back to 5 and repeat. Finish with a two minute cool down.

- *Interval training 20 minutes.* Ten minute warm up at moderate pace. Intervals every 20 seconds for five minutes. This means for 20 seconds go at an intensity of 6, then 20 seconds at intensity of 10, 20 seconds at 6, 20 seconds at 10, and so on for five minutes. Five minute cool down at moderate intensity. (This is tough and should only be done 3 times a week at the most. Intensity does not have to start at 6, pick a base and then bump it by 4 or 5)

> ### *Cardio Burns Fat!*
>
> I do my cardio right when I wake up, but to be honest with you, any cardio you do will be beneficial. If you are doing both one after another, lift first and then do the cardio. I have designed my lifting program to last around 45 to 50 minutes so it is pretty quick. The longest cardio you will be doing is 40 minutes so in total the longest you might spend in the gym is an hour and half. Not too bad considering you will have lifted and done cardio.

I believe also that you can and should have some fun with cardio, too. So I do at least two days of "fun cardio." Fun cardio is just what it sounds like. I like playing basketball, or football. Other options could be going for a bike ride, running, yoga, spinning, boxing class or whatever it is you like to do that is different than the active cardio. Whether you choose to do fun cardio is up to you, but it will not hinder the program, in fact it will be additional help in achieving desired results.

Acceptable Active Cardio Options

- Biking - whether on a stationary or recumbent bike, or outside, this is an excellent cardio option.

- Jogging or brisk walking (outside or treadmill) - Notice I say jogging, because running all out will only be used for the interval portion of your cardio.

- Swimming - Swimming is an unbelievable cardio workout, if you can do it, I suggest you give it a try.

- Elliptical Machine - This is my all-time favorite. It is easy and low to no impact; great if you have bad knees like me. I had my knee scoped and so this is the best thing I can do without causing pain to that area.

- Rowing machines – These are good too, just make sure your form is correct and you aren't putting undo stress on your back.

Tip: Fight Cardio Boredom

- Read your favorite magazine or novel (or you can even study) when doing long-duration cardio on stationary equipment like bikes, treadmills, elliptical machine. (You can purchase a slip on reading stand.)

- Place equipment within viewing distance of a TV.

- Bring music with you when walking or jogging.

- Do 20 minutes on one piece of equipment, then hop off and do another 20 minutes on another.

Aerobic Note – I know all about going out on Monday, and Tuesday nights. In fact, I am familiar with going out all nights of the week, but that's another story. My point is if you are going out all the time, you might actually be doing yourself a solid. That is, of course, if you aren't drinking like a fish and you are following the plan.

Going to clubs or bars with dance floors can actually be beneficial with regards to cardio. Now don't get me wrong . . . it is not a substitute for the designed active cardio options, BUT it can help to burn more calories!

So if you are one of those people who loves dancing and clubbing, go for it! **Just make sure you are paying strict attention to your diet while you are out.** Just because you go clubbing, does not mean you have to drink or eat crap. Be true to yourself and just enjoy being out. In fact look over at the bar, and think about all the crap everyone else is putting in their bodies, and then realize that you have a goal, and no one and nothing is going to get in your way of achieving it. Try these other fun cardio options as well, **football, basketball, soccer, baseball, softball, ultimate frisbee, swimming, tennis, golf etc.**

Chapter 9

Making It Real: The Secret to Partying and Not Ruining Your Diet

I've never been drunk, but often I've been over served. – George Gobel

OK, so we threw this party called the "Freezer" and it was amazing . . . but anyway, back to the original point of this book, which is not to promote my parties, but to shape your body and nutrition.

Parties (and restaurants/bars) aren't meant to be full of healthy and fun snacks . . . they are meant to have beer and liquor, and if there is food there, it is from the fridge of whoever is renting the house of where the party is happening (or it's fried appetizers from the bar . . . BAD CHOICE!). OK, so now that we know they are not the perfect setting for nutritious meals and drinks, let's take a look at what we can do to avoid the normal pitfalls of parties and bars.

> ***Not an undergrad?***
> Not a problem. Your parties may be different than those thrown by undergrads, but it's a good bet that there will be eating and drinking going on, so the "secret" to partying will still apply.

Stick to the Plan
First of all, you have got to follow the initial principles of the plan, even if it's a party day. So, basically that means you have been drinking plenty of water, you have eaten at least four times by the time of the party, hopefully five, and you have with you a nutrition bar or shake. (The bar is probably a better option since I imagine you'll be drinking other things.) Keep in mind I think the meal replacement bars and shakes I have approved (you can find them in the eating plan chapter) are great but not everyone can afford them or wants to use them. So any food found on the food guide is allowed at this time, just make sure you are eating something to stoke your metabolism into burning fat!

Now remember, you need at least 7 hours of sleep, and this is vital. So, if you are going out to a party and have class the next day, you must either pick a day where you have late classes, which would allow for the 7 hours, and or make sure that the next day you get at least one nap, but two is better. (Naps last for 45 minutes, no matter what anyone says about power naps . . . I say they need to be at least 45 minutes to an hour . . . 20 minutes only makes me more tired. Power naps are a crock of shit in my belief, no offense to all those power nappers.)

Somewhere about two to three hours after you ate last you should have the bar, whether you are inebriated or not . . . get that protein in your system. It will satiate you and keep your metabolism slightly moving.

Choose Wisely
OK, so you wanna have a beer or two or three. As long as it is your drinking day then that's fine, but try to choose the correct beer. Here are my favorites for what I call "nutritional drinking." (Catchy huh? Be careful. Im'a trademark it.)

1) Miller Light . . .bottom line, it's the best tasting light beer for my money.
2) Michelob Ultra . . . another good one nutritionally, but the taste's not the best if you ask me.
3) Bud Light . . . a proven winner, decent taste and decent nutritionally.
4) Other light beers are also good, so if you feel that others are better tasting, then go right ahead. I also like Sam Adams light, and Corona light. The idea is a light beer is better nutritionally.

So substitute any of these beers when playing beer pong, quarters, flip cup, or whatever new and fun games you have invented. I also understand that some of you beer connoisseurs hate light beer. Fine by me, go ahead and have your Guinness or Killians, I am simply saying light beer makes for a better option.

OK, now pay attention.
Here is the trick to drinking nutritionally. After every beer you drink, fill up the bottle with water and drink the water. This will add 16 ounces of water along with keeping you hydrated, PLUS water helps you feel full, so it may help to curb your hunger pains!! Now, if you think this might be embarrassing, I have a solution . . . go to the bathroom and fill the bottle there, or ask the bartenda' (if you're at a bar) for a cup of water and pour the water into the bottle. Embarrassing or not, you need to do it, especially if you hope to be shirtless, or be wearing a bikini in a few weeks.

At The Bar
Now if you are at a bar, the key is to have a beer in your hands whether you want to be drinking or not. Everyone knows that you feel a little out of place without something alcoholic in your hands. I know, 'cause I spent many nights with the same bottle of beer in my hand 4 hours after getting to the bar, but no one knew . . . anyway, everyone is too intoxicated to care . . . *so it comes down to whether you want to drink huge amounts or if you want to drink but also get buff.* Hey, small sacrifice. I'm not telling you *not to* drink – just modify your routine like this –

- If you do drink, twice a week is the limit. (However if you choose to drink twice then you have forfeited your fat meal for the week.)
- On the days you drink, your eating should be impeccable.
- If you're drinking beer, try to pick a light one.
- Match each alcoholic drink with a drink of water.

> ### *Fat Meals & Drink Days.*
> I do allow a **fat meal** and a **drink day** . . . Now, you are more than welcome to make them both drink days, or both fat meals, but if you choose to combine the two, then that is the limit for the week. If you choose two drink days, then you do not have the option for a fat meal. Same holds true for choosing two fat meals . . . no drink day then.

Liquor = Sugar
Now lets talk about liquor . . . I won't lie – I like Smirnoff Ice, I like Mike's Hard Lemonade, I like Twisted Tea, I like all those sugary drinks. My favorite drink of all time is an Amaretto sour . . . not a great nutritional drink. Now to be frank, these drinks will do more damage than the beer. You are more apt to drink these quicker and have more of them, so your calories skyrocket! Your insulin to a point, is controlled by your food and drink intake, will shoot straight through the roof courtesy of sugar and other high glycemic carbs. This is bad, really, really bad.

Those sugary drinks will be the death of you, so please if there is another option like BEER or wine, go with it. However, if you love Amaretto sours, like I do, or you are a die-hard margarita lover, then I might just have a solution for you. There is a certain company (Baja Bob's, see recipes section) who makes an excellent sour mix, margarita mix, bloody mary mix and others that are sugar free and low in calories. Ingenious if you ask me. Ahh, but here is the catch . . . each shot of liquor you put in each drink is roughly 100 calories, so the same rule applies here as with the beer –

- You finish one drink, you drink 16 ounces of water.
- I don't care how you do it, just do it!

If you are at a bar, then ask the bartenda' for a water with your drink and sip both and then refill the water and drink the glass of water before ordering or having another drink.

Most college kids have heard "Liquor before beer, you're in the clear. Beer before liquor, never sicker." Whether that's true or not, drinking the high sugar drink first does make sense.

- Drink the liquor drinks that might contain sugar first, so your body has a chance to continue to metabolize the sugar.

- Please don't drink those sugary drinks and then 2 minutes later go to sleep. This will greatly decrease your ability to get in shape, fit, ripped, and in a bikini or with your shirt off. Try to wait at least a half an hour before going to sleep.

Remember, I can't do it for you. You have to make some sacrifices, and so far, giving up sugary drinks doesn't seem like a big sacrifice to me!

One last tip. Don't play two-beer beer pong, play with one beer, or play with a partner so you aren't drinking as much, and have a water cup to sip from, and just call it a "chaser". "Chaser" is one of those words college kids love, so everyone will either accept that you need a chaser or think you're cool just for saying it.

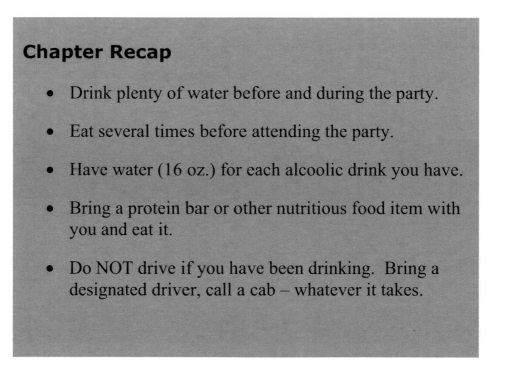

Chapter Recap

- Drink plenty of water before and during the party.

- Eat several times before attending the party.

- Have water (16 oz.) for each alcoolic drink you have.

- Bring a protein bar or other nutritious food item with you and eat it.

- Do NOT drive if you have been drinking. Bring a designated driver, call a cab – whatever it takes.

Chapter 10

HotBody FAQ's

How use doth breed a habit in a man! – William Shakespeare

Here I will answer questions I'm frequently asked. I will do my best to be as frank as possible, and I will try to touch on all concerns.

Q1 How long is the program, and do I have to be really, really strict on it? Or can I cheat on my diet a lot and skip my lifting for a few days.

A1 The main program is between 8 and 10 weeks (depending on your choice of schedule).
Yup, that's all . . . just 8 to 10 weeks. That means if you are planning a trip August 15th, then you need to start it by the middle of June or so. Not so bad if you ask me. As far as being really, really strict on it, here's the deal . . .

I don't believe that my program is that strict on its own, so that means that you have a lot less wiggle room. In fact, I have tried to make a program that allows you to be a COLLEGE KID (or busy person) and still reach the goals that you are hoping for. That means you can eat whatever you want at your fat meal and you can have alcohol once a week too! Hell, I even included tips on how to drink smarter! So the basic answer is, if you want to see the results that I saw, then yes, you must follow the program to a T.

Like I said, its only 8 to 10 weeks . . . but this doesn't mean you should stop the program, especially if you are seeing great results! This program is intended to be used for as long as you'd like to use it in order to seek good health! (And abs.)

Q2 How important is the nutrition portion relative to the other portions of your program?

A2 Seventy percent (that's 70%)! To see significant results you need to follow all portions of the program; however, the nutritional portion carries extra weight! You have to eat clean to look good. Bottom Line. So not paying attention to the nutritional portion will cause serious problems to your overall outcome. Lastly, the UP-DOWN carbohydrate role is there to help you burn more fat! So follow it.

Q3 If I am trying to gain some muscle instead of lose weight. Can I still use your program?

A3 A resounding *hell yea!* This program will help you add lean muscle mass, which can only help to burn body fat! You can't lose. The nutrition portion is geared towards gaining lean muscle mass, so once again, yes, this will work for you!

Q4 I am a girl and am worried about the effects that lifting weights will have on my feminine physique. I don't want to get too big.

A4 This is the most frequently asked question (and worry) from female clients. You will not get too big from this program. First, of all weight lifting is good for both men and women for benefits like heart health, increased lean muscle mass – and it flat out makes you more toned. Second, this program is only 8 or 10 ten weeks, and there is simply no way in that span of time you could get huge. This program is designed to get you in shape, not to make you a power lifter. As you know by now, lifting weights burns body fat.

Q5 I am a guy/girl who really likes to drink. Could I stretch the limit and add more days drinking if I go really hard on the weights and diet?

A5 NO. First let me say that drinking in moderation can be part of your diet (see Q1, above). Second, although I do know what it is like in college, and am fully aware you are going to partake in things that some might deem unhealthy, I in no way endorse binge drinking or the over- consumption of alcohol. Too much alcohol is a bad thing, people. I mean, come on now - give me a break. I have no say in what you do when you are not on my program, but if you want to see results on this program, you can't swap this part for that. I think the program is pretty lenient in that you can drink at all. Show me another legitimate best-selling program that says you can party and drink in moderation. . . exactly.

Q6 I am not in college. I am just looking for a program that will allow me to clean up my diet and get in shape. Can I use your program, or is it mainly just for the kid looking to go on spring break? Is it just a quick fix?

A6 Great question! Although I originally wrote this program from the standpoint of a kid who wants to get in shape quick for an event such as spring break while dealing with the college life, it really stands as a manual on how to get in shape for everyday people who are not very familiar with gyms or nutrition.

The Equipment Chapter (Chapter 5), for example, actually hits home for a lot of people. Any one who is unfamiliar with a gym and the machines will no doubt be hesitant to go in and try new exercises or start a weight-training program. You can't help but get healthier on this program. You can take any of the tips in the Cafeteria section (Chapter 3) and apply them to a restaurant and or to your own cooking at home. It's very simple.

No, this is not a quick fix. This is the diet I practice now and have been for the last three years. I have increased in strength and definition as well as lowered my cholesterol along the way. My body fat percentage has continued to drop and I feel energized upon waking up. So please, I encourage you to use the program for longer than ten weeks!

Q7 I thought eating a lot of carbs would make me fat? If this is true, then why do you include them in your diet section?

A7 The carbs I include in my diet section are <u>fat burners</u>. That's right - I believe they help in the fat burning process. I also use my UP-DOWN technique, which has given me incredible results in energy as well as burning fat. Your body needs carbs – they are your brains preferred fuel source. Take them away, and you're not doing so well in those 101 math or English classes! These carbs will not make you fat – in fact, they will do the exact opposite.

Q8 Should I eat before or after my workout, or both?

A8 Another great question! It is important to eat both times actually. Try to eat about a half hour before your workout, but keep the meal small, and include both protein and carbohydrates. The meal you consume after should also include both carbs and proteins, but should be a little bit more than the pre-workout meal.

Q9 Do I have to belong to a gym to take part in this program?

A9 No way! All you need is a few dumbbells and a bench that will act as both an incline an regular bench. If you are interested in purchasing gym equipment, then a great place to do so is Leisure Fitness!

Q10 If I miss a meal, cheat or mess up on a workout have I ruined my whole plan?

A10 Yes you have…JUST KIDDING! Of course not. No one is perfect; I know I'm not, not even close. I have missed workouts, and I have on occasion missed a meal or not eaten as healthy as I would have liked. Remember this program is not only meant for 8 or 10 weeks, but also for as long as you would like to have a "HotBody". If you fall off the wagon, then get your ass back up, and get back on. All I can ask is that you do your best, and try your hardest. Mistakes happen, it is whether you learn from them that is important. Question #1 talks about the need for discipline in this program, and that is true. But it would be foolish of me and anyone partaking in a program like this to think we would be perfect. No one is.

Q11 Will this program target my stomach for fat loss?

A11 Ahh, the million dollar question. The answer is yes and no. Yes it will target the fat on your stomach, but it will also target the fat on all of your body. You see, there is **no such thing** as spot reduction (where a certain section is the only place to lose fat). The only way to do this is liposuction, and despite the huge health risks that is, it is very expensive. This program however is not, and will help you to achieve a "hotbody" all over, not just in certain areas. I am often dumbfounded when I see diet programs that say they will target stomach fat. People please know, the only way to target fat is by doing so all over the body. Along these same lines, you can burn fat in <u>all</u> areas no matter what you have heard, even those that you think you can not. Areas like the stomach, the thighs, the ass…It doesn't matter; if you do the program you will burn the fat.

Q12 I hate doing anything aerobic, athletic, or basically anything that involves moving in the morning. Can I do my cardio later in the day?

A12 You may do your cardio whenever it works for you in your schedule. The idea is much along the lines of the Nike™ motto…"Just Do It!" Whether that is the morning, afternoon or evening is fine. All that I ask is that you do the cardio after you lift if you plan to do them at the same time. This will allow for more strength during lifting, and more fat burning during cardio. (I do my cardio in the morning so as to get that crap out of the way!)

Q13 I read and hear a lot about supplements for mass building and fat burning (i.e. diet pills), do you endorse these?

A13 I do not endorse any diet pills, nor do I think that super-duper supplements that promise fat loss and muscle gain are needed on this program. Protein, a multi-vitamin and possibly some type of good fat (CLA or other essential fatty acids) are all that I think are needed.

Chapter 11

I Wanna Hear From You!

The reward of a thing well done is to have done it. – *Ralph Waldo Emerson*

Well, there ya have it. This is the program that got me the results I wanted, and it included all my favorites (Outback Steakhouse visits, hot wings, beer, liquor, etc.) - in moderation. I am certain that if you follow the plan it will no doubt work wonders for you. You will be comfortable shirtless (guys) or in a bikini (gals) in no time flat! I think the best thing about this whole plan is that you can follow it way past college. It can be incorporated into a daily life for just about anyone and everyone.

Not an undergrad?
Got a 9 to 5 job? No biggy, this plan will work. Work nights? No problem, it works there too. Been out of college for 20 years? Not a problem, the basics of this program can work for you as well.

OK, now I need <u>your</u> help. Any good trainer will want to know what's working and what's not for his or her clients. I need you to tell me what about the program you liked best and what about it you flat out hated. How's it working for you? Are you planning to stay on it beyond your initial goal period?

So I'm asking you to write to me . . . whether you want to tell me that my program sucks or that you think my recipes are horrible or phenomenal. Maybe you want to tell me how your school throws better parties than mine. Or maybe, just maybe, you want to tell me that with this program you have achieved noticeable results not only for your body, but for your mind as well. I also would love to hear your recipes that you have created, and if I think they are good I will put them in future editions of the book!

Here's where to reach me: HotBody101MK@hotmail.com

Also, please visit the website! www.**HotBody101.com**

I can only hope that you will be as pleased with my program as I myself and my clients have been. Anyway, whatever you want to tell me, please do it! You see I'm just a regular guy, probably a lot like you. I had make-ups and break-ups, went out the night before tests, I stayed up nights to write papers and slept days, I went on road trips, I played midnight basketball!

I'm with ya'll! I did it too, and I just want you guys to know that you <u>can</u> make a huge change in your body and gain confidence in a short period. Remember, I started out at 26% body fat (I'm now at 7%), so I know the woes of going to the beach and not taking off my shirt. I've been there. In fact, <u>you</u> may be starting from a better beginning point than I did – and in 8 to 10 weeks, you can be **a lot** better than you are now.

OK, I'm done rambling now. Here's just one last request that you let me know how this program works for you. Thanks so much for your time, and best of luck with the program (not with the girl or guy you meet tonight at the bar ☺) . . . well I guess him or her too . . .

Appendix 1

Recipes
Low cal, low sugar food and good drinks too!

Once you start paying attention to the food you are eating, you might even get into making more complex dishes. When that happens, scope out recipes online or better yet, think about purchasing a cookbook that works for you. For now, here are some very quick and easy "recipes" that work with The Program.

Couple of quick notes: Chicken breasts should be trimmed of all visible fat. Feel free to substitute ½ cup shredded fat free cheese for one piece sliced fat free cheese.

Food Recipes
These recipes can and should be used in the diet program! They all include approximate numbers of calories, carbohydrates, and protein so there is no guess work for your food journal.

TIP: Grilling is a quick, healthy and tasty way to cook up your meats. I've found that the George Forman Grill ™ works great and is easy to use. You can also broil in the oven or grill/sauté in a frying pan using Pam cooking spray or a small amount of olive oil.

Plain Ol' Oatmeal

- ½ cup oatmeal
- 1 cup water

1 min 45 sec in microwave on high, let sit a minute. Enjoy. (150 cals. 30 carbs. Negligible protein)

Cinnamon Oatmeal
Plain ol' oatmeal (1/2 cup), sprinkle on some cinnamon. Very tasty. (150 cals. 30 carbs. Negligible protein)

Breakfast Egg-n-Cheese Pita

- One whole wheat pita
- 6 egg whites
- 1 slice fat free cheese
- ½ cup onions chopped
- pepper

Scramble egg whites with cheese and onion. Season with pepper. Spoon into pita. Enjoy. (305 cals. 30 carbs. 25 grams protein)

Mike's Spicy-n-Cheesy Egg White Omelet

- 6 egg whites
- 1 slice fat free cheese
- half tomato, cut up in small sections
- ½ cup onions
- ½ cup red/yellow/orange or green pepper
- Cholula ™ sauce (or your favorite hot sauce)

Heat pan, use Pam instead oil. Beat eggs, pour into hot pan, use spatula to pull cooking egg to one side of pan while tilting pan to let loose egg drip back to open spot in pan. Add in all other ingredients. Cover and reduce heat to allow to cook through (couple of minutes). Fold in half as you empty onto the plate. (275 cals. 5 carbs. 30 grams protein)

Scrambled Cheese Eggs

- 4 egg whites
- 1 whole egg
- 1 slice fat free cheese or ½ cup shredded fat free cheese
- pepper

Use a whisk to mix up the eggs if you have one. It works great. If not, use a fork and some good wrist action to get some air in there. Scramble in the cheese after the eggs begin to cook. (210 cals. 5 carbs. 20 grams protein)

Cafeteria Grilled Chicken Salad

- Grilled chicken breast
- Garden salad (romaine lettuce, green or other pepper, cucumbers, carrots, etc.)
- Balsamic vinegar

Slice the grilled chicken breast into the garden salad. Add a little balsamic vinegar – a serving size! Enjoy! (300 cals. Negligible carbs. 30 grams protein)

Cheesy Turkey Dogs

- 2 fat free turkey dogs
- 1 slice fat free cheese
- 1 whole grain or wheat hot dog roll.

Line roll with cheese, place dogs on roll. Close and wrap the whole thing in a paper towel. Microwave to heat dogs and melt cheese (about 20 seconds).
(375 cals. 30 carbs. 30 grams protein)

Cheesy, Tangy Turkey Burger

- 6 ounces lean ground turkey, 99% fat free (usually says 1% fat on label)
- 1 slice fat free cheese
- ½ cup onions
- 1 teaspoon barbeque sauce

Mix turkey and sauce, form into patty, grill, put on cheese just before done. Enjoy on one whole grain roll. (350 cals. 40 carbs. 30 grams protein)

Serious Grilled Chicken

- 1 chicken breast
- garlic powder and pepper
- McCormick Grillmates (Roasted Garlic or Montreal Chicken) seasoning

Season chicken with all ingredients. Grill on barbeque or in frying pan with a little Pam or olive oil. (300 cals. Negligible carbs. 30 grams protein)

Even More Serious Grilled Chicken

- 1 chicken breast
- garlic powder and pepper
- crushed hot pepper
- McCormick Grillmates Salt Free Chicken Seasoning
- tablespoon mustard

Mix seasonings and mustard, paint chicken, grill chicken. Grill on barbeque or in frying pan with a little Pam or olive oil. (300 cals. Negligible carbs. 30 grams protein)

Garlic Broiled Chicken

- 1 chicken breast, halved, skinned
- ½ tsp. garlic, minced
- 1 tbsp. fresh lemon juice
- 1 tsp. Dijon mustard
- ½ tsp. salt, seasoned salt or salt-free seasoning
- fresh ground black pepper

Combine all ingredients for basting sauce in small bowl. Brush over chicken. Broil for 10 minutes each side, 2 inches from heat, brushing frequently with sauce. (300 cals. Negligible carbs. 30 grams protein)

Grilled Cheesy Chicken

- 1 chicken breast
- garlic powder and pepper
- McCormick Grillmates Salt Free Chicken Seasoning
- 1 slice fat free cheese

Season chicken, grill, apply cheese with a minute or two to go to allow melting. Enjoy. ((330 cals. 5 carbs. 35 grams protein)

Grilled Chicken Cheese Steak

- 1 chicken breast
- garlic powder
- pepper
- McCormick grillmates Salt free Chicken Seasoning
- one slice fat free cheese
- one teaspoon fat free mayo

Season and grill chicken, chop chicken and stuff into wheat pita with cheese and mayo. (400 cals. 40 carbs. 35 grams protein)

Whole Wheat Steak Fajitas

- 1 whole wheat fajita
- 8 ounce flank steak
- McCormick Grillmates steak seasoning
- 1 tablespoon garlic powder
- 1 tablespoon pepper

Cook steak with seasoning on the grill or in a pan with PAM cooking spray – Slice thin and put into a whole wheat pita. Add any vegetables desired. (410 cals. 30 carbs. 40 grams protein)

Whole Wheat Chicken Fajitas

- 1 whole wheat fajita
- 1 large chicken breast
- McCormick Grillmates chicken seasoning
- 1 tablespoon garlic powder
- 1 tablespoon pepper
- Veggies (your choice)

Cook chicken with seasoning on the grill or in a pan with PAM cooking spray. Slice thin and put into a whole wheat pita. Add any vegetables desired. (390 cals. 30 carbs. 30 grams protein)

"Some Good Ass Steak"
(The name comes from people trying it and saying… "Man, that is some good ass steak!")

- 6 ounces top sirloin
- pepper
- garlic powder
- ½ cup barbeque sauce
- McCormick Grillmates steak seasoning

Season steak, grill, apply sauce at very end of grilling. (400cals. 10 carbs. 40 grams protein)

Plain Ol' Turkey Burgers

- 24 ounces lean ground turkey
- 99% fat free (usually says 1% fat on label)
- ½ cup bottled southwest salsa or other flavor salsa
- pepper

Mix turkey and salsa, form into 4 patties, season, grill. You can eat one for dinner and store the other three in the 'fridge for other meals during the week. (270 cals. 20 carbs. 30 grams protein) (*A slice of fat free cheese adds roughly 35 cals. 5 carbs. And 4 grams of protein.*)

Turkey Burger Chili

- 24 ounces lean ground turkey
- 99% fat free (usually says 1% fat on label)
- ½ cup onion
- ½ cup green pepper
- ½ cup red pepper
- ½ cup sliced jalapeño peppers
- 1 tablespoon hot sauce

Cook turkey meat first (with PAM cooking spray) then add ingredients and cook for five minutes – Serve in a mug. (300 cals. 15 carbs. 30 grams protein)

Turkey Burger Chili Sloppy Joes

- 24 ounces lean ground turkey
- 99% fat free (usually says 1% fat on label)
- ½ cup onion
- ½ cup green pepper
- ½ cup red pepper
- ½ cup sliced jalapeño peppers
- 1 tablespoon hot sauce

Cook turkey meat first (with PAM cooking spray) then add ingredients and cook for five minutes. Put one serving (roughly the size of a fist) in a whole wheat bun and enjoy! (400 cals. 45 carbs. 30 grams protein)

Tasty Turkey Meatloaf

- 1 pound and a half ground extra-lean turkey breast
- 1 large onion
- ½ cup bread crumbs (use wheat bread and make your own!)
- 2 tablespoons Dijon Mustard
- 2 egg whites
- 2 cloves garlic finely chopped

Heat oven to 375, and spray loaf pan with cooking spray (like PAM) Mix all the ingredients together and then bake for about an hour uncovered – When no longer pink in the center or the temp. is 160 degrees, it is done. It makes 6 servings, so slice it into six pieces, and eat one for a meal!) (250 cals. 15 carbs. 30 grams protein)

Boca Burger Chili Sloppy Joes (Meat Free)

- 2 servings of Boca Burger ground burger
- ½ cup onion
- ½ cup green pepper
- ½ cup red pepper
- ½ cup sliced jalapeño peppers
- ½ cup chopped mushrooms
- 1 tablespoon hot sauce

Cook Boca Burger meat first in pan with Pam cooking spray, then add vegetables and let cook for 5 minutes – let simmer – Put contents in a whole wheat bun and enjoy! (320 cals. 45 carbs. 22 grams protein)

Lemon Dill Salmon with a Touch of Garlic

- 16 ounces of salmon
- ½ cup lemon juice
- ½ cup lime juice
- 1 teaspoon garlic
- 1 tablespoon dill
- ½ cup extra virgin olive oil

Mix all ingredients minus the fish together. Use the ingredients as a marinade and spread all over fish. Let sit for 15 minutes then cook on grill. (8 ounce serving is 320 cals. negligible carbs. 35 grams protein, give the other serving to your significant other)

Balsamic Vinaigrette Tuna with Healthy Stir-Fry Snow Peas

- 1 large tuna steak, roughly 8 to 10 ounces
- ½ cup balsamic vinaigrette
- ½ cup lemon juice
- ½ cup lime juice
- 1 tablespoon extra virgin olive oil

Tuna should be cooked on the grill while the snow peas are simmering on the stove (cook them with PAM cooking spray). Mix ingredients together and use ¾ as a marinade for the tuna and the other ¼ should be put into the pan with the snow peas. Combine snow peas and tuna and enjoy your five star meal. (375 cals. 10 carbs. 50 grams of protein)

Your Recipes

_____

_____

_____

_____

_____

_____

_____

DRINK RECIPES

These are designed for a drink day only! I have tried to make them as healthy as possible, but I have also included some of my favorite drinks because I like them and I think you will too! If you are 21 years of age that is...(As a side note I was and am a bartenda' so I enjoy making drinks, but I can not stress enough the need for responsible drinking.)

Drinks With Alcohol

Bay Breeze

- 1 oz. vodka
- pineapple juice
- cranberry juice
- Ice

Fill with equal parts Pineapple Juice and Cranberry Juice and ice.

Bloody Mary

- 1 oz. vodka
- 3 drops Tabasco sauce
- 3 drops Worcestershire
- ½ tablespoon salt
- ½ tablespoon pepper

Fill with tomato juice and add a celery stick.

Chocolate Cake Shot

- Lemon flavored vodka
- Frangelico

Combine all equal parts.

Dreamsicle (Low Sugar Version)

- 1 oz. 43 Liqueur
- ½ oz Triple Sec

Fill with Baja Bob's sugar free sweet-n-sour mix.

Fire Ball Shot

- Cinnamon Schnapps
- 2 drops of Tabasco sauce

Combine all equal parts.

Fuzzy Navel

- 1 oz. peach schnapps

Fill with orange juice and ice.

Gin and Tonic

- 1 oz. gin (I like Tanqueray)
- tonic water
- ice

Combine in tall glass. Add wedge of lime if desired.

Grasshopper (Low Fat Version)

- ¾ oz. green crème de menthe
- ¾ oz. light crème de cacao
- 1 ½ oz. fat free milk (skim)

Combine and enjoy.

Hairy Navel

- ½ oz. vodka
- ½ oz. peach schnapps

Fill with orange juice and ice.

Kamikaze Shot

- vodka
- Triple Sec
- lime juice

Combine all equal parts.

Long Island Iced Tea (Mikes Low Sugar Version)

- ½ oz. Vodka
- ½ oz. Gin
- ½ oz. Rum
- ½ oz. Tequila

Combine ingredients and fill with diet coke and 2 ounces Baja Bob's sugar free sweet-n-sour mix. Serve with ice.

Low Sugar Pina Colada

- 1 oz. rum
- 4 oz. Baja Bob's crazy caribe pina colada mix
- 4 ice cubes
- 2 oz. of water

Blend all ingredients. Enjoy.

Maitai (Low Sugar Version)

- 1 oz. rum
- ½ oz. Amaretto
- ½ oz. Triple Sec

Combine ingredients and fill with Baja Bob's sugar free sweet-n-sour mix.

Melon Ball Shot

- Vodka
- Melon Liqueur
- Pineapple Juice

Combine all equal parts.

Mike's Mimosa

1 ½ oz. of your favorite wine mixed with 2 ½ ounces Baja Bob's sugar free sweet-n-sour mix.

OBX Frozen Punchless Punch

- 1 oz. Amaretto
- 8 oz. Baja Bob's sugar free sweet-n-sour mix
- 8 ice cubes
- half an orange
- half a banana
- ½ cup OJ
- 1/2 cup fat free milk

Blend all ingredients - trust me, it's good.

OBX Unfrozen Punchless Punch

- 1 shot Amaretto
- 8 oz. Baja Bob's sugar free sweet-n-sour mix
- 4 ice cubes
- ½ cup OJ
- ½ cup Skim Milk

Blend all ingredients.

Orgasm Shot

- Vodka
- Kahlua
- Amaretto
- Skim Milk

Combine all equal parts.

Pink Squirrel (low fat)

- ¾ oz. crème de almond
- ¾ oz. light crème de cacao
- 1 ½ oz. skim milk

Shake with ice and then strain into short glass.

Rum and Diet Coke

- 1 oz. rum

Fill with diet coke and ice.

Rum Runner (Mikes Low Sugar Version)

- 1 oz. rum
- ½ oz. banana liqueur
- ½ oz. apricot liqueur

Fill with Baja Bob's sugar free sweet-n-sour mix – Serve over ice

Screwdriver

- 1 oz. vodka

Fill with orange juice.

Seven and Seven

- 1 oz. Seagram's Seven

Fill with diet Seven-Up and ice.

Sex on the Beach

- ½ oz. black raspberry liquor
- ½ oz. melon liqueur

Fill with pineapple juice. Shake with ice and then strain.

Sugar Free Amaretto and Cream

- 1 oz. Amaretto
- 4 oz. Baja Bob's sugar free sweet-n-sour mix
- 2 oz. water
- 4 ice cubes
- ½ cup skim milk

Mix all ingredients.

Sugar Free Amaretto Sour

- 1 oz. Amaretto
- 4 ounces Baja Bob's sugar free sweet-n-sour mix
- 2 ounces water
- 4 ice cubes

Mix all ingredients.

Sugar Free Margarita

- 1 oz. tequila
- 4 oz. Baja Bob's margarita mix
- 4 ice cubes
- 2 oz. water

Mix all ingredients.

Sugar Free SoCo Sour

- 1 oz. Southern Comfort
- 4 oz. Baja Bob's sugar free sweet-n-sour mix
- 2 oz. water
- 4 ice cubes

Mix all ingredients. Garnish with lime.

Sugar Free Whiskey Sour

- 1 oz. whiskey
- 4 oz. Baja Bob's sugar free sweet-n-sour mix
- 2 oz. water
- 4 ice cubes

Mix all ingredients

Tequila Sunrise

- 1 oz. Tequila

Fill with orange juice and a ½ cup of Grenadine.

Vodka Tonic

- 1 oz. vodka (I like Grey Goose)

Fill with tonic water and ice.

Drinks With No Alcohol

Most drinks can be made non-alcoholic for the under 21 crowd and they will taste great. Below I have put the three most difficult to mix.

Mock Mimosa

- 1 cup white grape juice, chilled
- ¾ cup orange juice, chilled
- ½ cup club soda, chilled
- 2 orange slices for garnish

In a pitcher or other container, combine juices, mix. Pour into two glasses. Pour half the club soda into each glass. Cut halfway through each orange slice and use to garnish each glass.

Mock Margaritas

- 1 can (12 oz.) frozen lemonade concentrate, thawed, undiluted
- 1 can (12 oz.) frozen limeade concentrate, thawed, undiluted
- 1 cup confectioners' sugar
- 6 cups finely crushed ice
- green food color (optional)
- 1 bottle (1 liter) club soda, chilled
- lime slices
- coarse salt

In 4-quart non-metal container, combine lemonade, limeade, sugar, ice – mix well. Cover and freeze, stirring occasionally. Remove container from freezer about 30 minutes before serving, let stand at room temperature to thaw slightly. To serve: for each drink, spoon about 2 cups of the "slush" into electric blender container, add 1 cup soda, cover and blend. Rub rim of glass with lime slice and dip rim in course salt. Fill glass and enjoy. Makes about 12 1-cup servings.

Virgin Bloody Mary

- 3 drops Tabasco sauce
- 3 drops Worcestershire
- ½ tablespoon salt
- ½ tablespoon pepper

Fill with tomato juice and add a celery stick

SMOOTHIES AND SUCH . . .

These Smoothies and shakes are not permitted on the diet, however, if you really want to stay healthy but are craving something that tastes great, these are the great options! They are not terrible nutritionally, but they do have a bit too many calories and carbs and not enough protein, so save them for a "fat" -- which then would become a healthy fat / cheat day (go figure). You can also add some protein powder to these drinks to give you a protein boost even on a "fat day."

Banana-Orange Shake

- 1 ripe large banana, peeled and sliced
- 1 ripe medium orange, peeled and cut into chunks
- ½ cup skim milk
- 2 scoops vanilla frozen yogurt
- 1 teaspoon vanilla (if you have it)

In blender combine everything and blend until smooth. Serve immediately. Makes about 2 1-cup servings. An unlimited number of fruit combinations is possible! Try strawberry-peach, papaya-mango, banana-melon.

Yogurt and Oat Dazzler

- ¾ cup old-fashioned or quick-cooking rolled oats, uncooked
- 1 cup low-fat or skim milk
- 1 ripe banana, peeled and cut into chunks
- 1 cup low-fat or non-fat coffee yogurt

In blender, blend oats until they become a powder. Add milk, banana and yogurt to oat powder in blender. Blend 20 seconds or until smooth. Serve immediately. Makes about 3 1-cup servings. Delicious for breakfast and has potassium and calcium.

Apricot-Pineapple-Strawberry Protein Fruit Smoothie

- ¼ cup crushed pineapple (canned, get it in it's own juice instead of syrup)
- 1 fresh apricot, diced
- 6 strawberries
- ½ banana
- ¾ cup skim milk
- ¾ cup water
- 1 heaping tbsp. high-quality protein powder (optional)
- 1 tsp. flax seed oil (optional)

Blend until thoroughly mixed and serve immediately. Serves 1.

Chocolate - Strawberry - Raspberry Dream

- 8 oz. skim milk
- 5 raspberries
- 1 ¼ cup crushed ice
- 1 cup nonfat frozen chocolate yogurt
- 6 strawberries
- 1 tsp. flax seed oil (optional)

Blend until thoroughly mixed and serve immediately. Serves 1.

Peanut Butter - Banana Swirl Smoothie

- 8 oz. skim milk
- ¼ cup natural peanut butter
- 1 cup nonfat frozen yogurt
- 1 ¼ cup crushed ice
- half banana
- 1 tsp. flax seed oil (optional)

Blend until thoroughly mixed and serve immediately. Serves 1.

Valentines Smoothie

- 8 oz. skim milk
- 6 strawberries
- 1 cup nonfat frozen vanilla yogurt
- 1 ¼ cup crushed ice

In container of electric blender, process fruit and the rest of ingredients. Blend until thoroughly mixed and serve immediately. Serves 1.

Creamsicle Smoothie

- 6 oz. orange juice
- 1/3 cup nonfat frozen yogurt vanilla
- ½ cup peaches
- ½ banana
- 1 ¼ cup crushed ice

Blend fruit and the rest of ingredients. Blend until thoroughly mixed and serve immediately. Serves 1.

Summer Lovin' Smoothie

- 1 ¾ cups seedless watermelon
- 1 tablespoon honey
- ½ kiwi
- 1 ¼ cup crushed ice

In container of electric blender, process fruit and the rest of ingredients. Blend until thoroughly mixed and serve immediately. Serves 1.

Pina Colada Smoothie

- 1 cup nonfat regular yogurt
- ½ banana
- ½ cup pineapple
- 1 cup skim milk
- ½ cup chopped coconut
- 1 ¼ cup crushed ice

In container of electric blender, process fruit and the rest of ingredients. Blend until thoroughly mixed and serve immediately. Serves 1.

Your Recipes

_____

_____

_____

_____

_____

_____

Again, here is the deal with smoothies…

Basically you can throw any type of fruit in there and mix it with yogurt and ice and have a great tasting drink. So try your own recipes and if you find some that you think are great, send them along to me for inclusion in the next edition of the HotBody or posting on the website (www.hotbody101.com). You will be properly credited!

Keep in mind that although these seem healthy, there are hidden fats and huge amounts of sugar we don't need and aren't allowed during the diet portion of the program, so save them for a somewhat healthy treat during your fat meal. Despite not being allowed during the normal diet portion of the program, they make a great alternative to the five pieces of cheesecake or ten snickers bars you might choose, yet it is up to you.

_____

_____

_____

_____

_____

_____

Appendix 2

The New (and Improved) Food Pyramid

You are what you eat…

This is my idea of what the food pyramid should look like. I don't believe that 11 servings of high glycemic carbs (currently acceptable on the USDA charge) is the way to a lean body. Just my opinion. This "new and improved" pyramid has been a basic guideline to my eating routine.

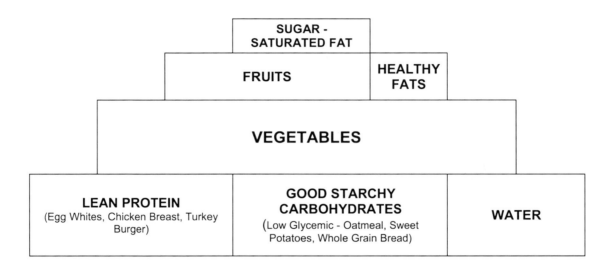

Appendix 3

Glossary

My terms and common terms.

Aerobic Exercise. Any activity involving large muscles, done for an extended period of time. Aerobic exercise helps achieve weight loss, but it also provides cardiovascular benefits. Examples of aerobic exercise include walking, biking, jogging, elliptical machine, swimming, aerobic classes, cross-country skiing, etc.

Bartenda'. Bartender just spelled cooler.

Bigz. My Dad and biggest supporter. (Also a user of the program, and a vegetarian who had no problem adjusting his meals without the meat.) Reading and rereading drafts is not fun, but my dad persevered. I owe him many thanks for not only proofing, but also being a guinea pig with regards to the program. He completed it and now is thinner, more toned, and feeling great! He was also the person whom I first approached about my idea for this book, and to my surprise he just said, "Let's do it!" And so we have…

Body Composition Test. A test used to determine the current percentage of body fat a person has.

Body Mass Index (BMI). A popular method used to gauge whether or not a person is overweight. BMI is calculated by dividing a person's weight (in kilograms) by his or her height (in meters, squared).

Caf. See "commons"

Calorie. A unit of measure for the amount of energy released when the body breaks down food.

Cambered bar. That crooked looking bar that people use for curls.

Carbohydrate. Any of a large group of sugars, starches, cellulose and gums that the body uses by converting into glucose, a simple sugar, for fuel.

Carbs. Carbohydrates

Cholesterol. A type of fat that circulates in your blood. It comes from two sources. The body makes its own regardless of what is eaten and from foods containing animal products.

CLA. Conjugated Linoleic Acid. A naturally occurring free fatty acid. In some studies it has been shown to reduce fat, and promote muscle tone. CLA is an unsaturated fat, and can be found mainly in meat and dairy products.

Clean food. Food that is not processed, and is free of hydrogenation and or other processes, which try to add shelf life.

Commons. My cafeteria at Salisbury University.

Courtney. The female model, who is one of the most fit girls I know! Her phone number is…just kidding ☺

Concentric. The lifting portion of an exercise.

Eccentric. The lowering portion of an exercise.

Fat meals. Anything you imagine them to be. (YES, even cheese fries…starting to see a pattern?)

Fat. Organic compounds that are made up of carbon, hydrogen, and oxygen, it is the body's most concentrated source of energy. Like protein and carbohydrates, fat is a principal and essential component of the diet.

Fibrous. Vegetables that contain fiber. Ex. Broccoli

"Get fit" gene. Also known as the "get ripped" gene in some cultures. This gene is a fictional gene that allows the person to be born with all the knowledge in the world about getting fit, and the equipment to use in the gym. (Tell you what, the only gene I know is my boy, Jean. He goes to school at Virginia Tech . . . but I digress . . .)

High Glycemic Carbs. Causes insulin levels to jump, which can promote fat storage . . . (Bad carbs)

High Protein Diet. Diets that recommend receiving up to 30% of calories (or more) from protein as opposed to the recommended 10%-15% from protein. These diets also recommend low carbohydrate consumption and are often high in total fat. (Although we will take in a higher amount of protein than other diets, I hate to call it a high protein diet, since we do not limit our carbs, and our fat does not increase.)

Jodie. My Mom (and editor)! Quite an amazing job she has done in helping me. Any of you who either relate to 24 hour workdays and or have parents who never stop working can appreciate my mom. She keeps my family on track, and in fact made this book a reality. Her editing skills are of the highest quality, and her knowledge of not only the computer but its applications continuously leaves me in awe. Thanks mom.

Jungle juice. Come on now, I'm not going to promote drinking . . . well . . . . nah

LobLolly Girls. These girls were the ones who introduced me to "Jungle Juice". They are, Puma, Sharon, (honorary Loblolly girls) Arden, Meredith, Jaime, Lil' Kristen, and Lauren.

Low Glycemic Carbs. Carbs that burn slowly and give you a prolonged amount of energy . . . (Good carbs)

Metabolism. The amount of energy (calories) your body burns to maintain itself. Metabolism is the process in which nutrients are acquired, transported, used and disposed of by the body.

Monounsaturated fat. A type of fat found in large amounts in foods from plants, including olive, peanut and canola oil.

Overhand grip. The grip you would use to push a lawn mower.

Peeps. Parents, whether they are yours or mine . . . . ex. "-My peeps are awesome!" Or "Your peeps are awesome!"

Pete. My other roommate, who also went to the gym with us (Riggzz and I) for a good part of our junior and senior years. Pete and I made many trips to TCBY ™ for non-fat no sugar added frozen yogurt. (Which can and should be consumed during your fat meal for a better option than ice cream)

Polyunsaturated Fat. A type of fat that is found in large amounts in foods from plants, including safflower, sunflower and corn oil.

Protein. An organic compound that is the "building block" of the human body. Protein builds and maintains muscle tissue.

Recommended Daily Allowance (RDA). The level of essential nutrients required to adequately meet the known nutrient needs of practically all healthy persons, according to the Food and Nutrition Board of the National Academy of Sciences.

Riggzz. My roommate and one my best friends in college and in my life. This is the kid that went with me to the gym everyday . . . thanx man, I owe you more than you know. Rami also did the program and went from a super skinny 130, to a solid and ripped 150 in about ten weeks. To this day he still is making great improvements, and is still the best training partner around!

Salisbury University. The place where my body transformation began. It is nestled on the Eastern Shore of Maryland.

Sarah. The amazing person that I complained and vented too, all the while she sat with a patient ear listening and giving excellent advice. Knowing she would always lend an ear and advice was vital in the programs completion. From the bottom of my heart, thank you...MTW (She also happens to be an excellent dancer!)

Saturated Fat. A type of fat most often found in animal food products including milk, eggs, meat and butter. Saturated fat is also found in vegetable products such as coconut and palm oil. Studies show that too much saturated fat in a person's diet increases heart disease risk.

Seth. My bro (for real, biological brother). Also used this program two years ago and went from 280 pounds to 225 pounds all the while dropping a good 10% of body fat in 8 weeks. Seth also was a huge help in the planning and later editing process. I am proud of his accomplishments and owe him thanks for all the technical help!

Snacky. The act of eating too much and or feeling ridiculously full . . . ex. "I am so friggin snacky, I just ate five pounds of hot wings".

Spinning. Cycling class.

"Throw up" weight. How much weight you have lifted.

Undergrad. A college student in undergraduate school.

Underhand grip. Your clenched fist (palms) face the sky

University of Maryland. Although this University does not really play a role in the book, I would just like to say that everyone should be a Terps fan! **GO TERPS**!!

Wheels. 45 pound plates.

Appendix 4
References and Recommendations

The ***HotBody.101 Diet and Exercise Program*** is the product of my own personal improvement efforts. As you would expect, I did a lot of reading (books and magazines) and visiting online sites in my "self-help" phase. I have woven this research and my training (NESTA certification) and personal experience into this program. Here are the sites and publications that directly impacted this program – some of which are sited directly in the text, and others that I believe you may find interesting or useful.

ONLINE

LifeClinic Nutrition/Fitness – online nutrition and fitness [http://www.lifeclinic.com/focus/nutrition/]. The section about reading the food label is largely from this site [http://www.lifeclinic.com/focus/nutrition/food-label.asp]. This site offers an excellent presentation of nutrition facts and "look ups" – a great reference when you start building your own menus and want to evaluate the nutritive value of your foods.

U.S. Department of Agriculture – USDA [http://www.usda.gov]. While I don't agree with the USDA food pyramid, this site does offer a lot of information and useful PDF downloads.

[http://www.collegedrinkingprevention.gov] – This website provided many useful and important facts about the dangers of alcohol.

I visited lots of sites for Smoothie recipes. I've noticed that some are no longer "found" – so I'd suggest you just type "Smoothie" into your favorite search engine if you are looking for smoothie recipes. You'll find a wealth of healthy recipes searching the internet this way. Don't assume you can add a meal because it looks "healthy" to you. There is a method to the plan, and sticking to the Food Chart is critical for success in 8 to 10 weeks.

MAGAZINES

Muscle & Fitness presents Total Nutrition (July 2003). There is a blizzard of fitness magazines out there. I believe *Muscle & Fitness* magazine is one of the best. I read it regularly for factual information, new ideas, motivation and recipes. Their Total Nutrition publication provided ideas for some of my recipes ideas. "Find Healthy Fast-Food Choices" is from this publication directly.

Other magazines that have contributed to my approach and I highly recommend, in addition to *Muscle & Fitness*, are: *Men's Health, Men's Fitness, Muscle & Fitness Hers, Muscle Media, Optimum Lifestyle, Fitness Rx,* and *Flex.*

BOOKS

Body for Life, Bill Phillips and Michael D'Orso. New York: HarperCollins Publishers, 1999. This has been on the New York Times Bestseller List, and for good reason – it's inspiring! I think Bill Phillips is a great advocate for a healthy and nutritious way of living. I like this plan, but feel that the carbohydrate manipulation and different cardio / aerobic options in the **HotBody.101** plan may help to burn fat quicker.

Food Fight, Kelly D. Brownell, PhD. and Katherine Battle Horgen, Ph.D. Chicago: McGraw-Hill, 2004. Described as "the inside story of the food industry, America's obesity crisis, and what we can do about it," this book is a real eye opener.

The South Beach Diet, Arthur Agatston, MD. Rodale, Inc., 2003. There has been such a buzz with this book, I felt it important to read. The book is about two-thirds recipes – and some of them look pretty good. It is very food centered. There is not much in the sense of strength training for fat burning purposes in this book. This seems to be more about losing weight than it is about getting toned and fit. Yet it is a nice place to start if you are looking for good recipes! Most require some work in the kitchen, so the ease of them may be limited.

The World's Fittest You, Joe Decker, Dutton Books, Jan 2004. This book is an excellent tool for weight management, physical fitness, and anything to do with overall health. Joe is and will continue to be a mentor of mine and I encourage anyone who enjoyed my book to check his out as well.

Appendix 5 EXERCISE CHART – 10 Week (copy and use for your own, or email me for the Excel file)

10 WEEK PROGRAM

Exercise	Sets*	Reps	Week 1 (date)	Week 2 (date)	Week 3 (date)	Week 4 (date)	Week 5 (date)	Week 6 (date)	Week 7 (date)	Week 8 (date)	Week 9 (date)	Week 10 (date)
Monday - Chest, Back, Calves, and Abs												
#1 Incline dumbbell chest press	4	12-10-10-8										
#2 Flat bench dumbbell press	4	12-10-10-8										
#3 Flyes	4	12-10-10-8										
#4 Wide grip pull down	4	12-10-10-8										
#5 One arm dumbbell row	4	12-10-10-8										
#6 Leg ups	4	12-10-10-8										
#7 Crunch on the floor	4	30-25-20-15										
#8 Standing calf (biggest textbook or step)	4	16-14-12-10										
Wednesday - Shoulders, Straps, Hamstrings, Abs												
#1 Dumbbell press	4	12-10-10-8										
#2 Dumbbell rear shoulder raise	4	12-10-10-8										
#3 Upright rows or side lateral raises (your choice)	4	12-10-10-8										
#4 Dumbbell forward shoulder raise	4	20-10-10-8										
#5 Crunch on the floor (really try to feel the squeeze)	4	30-25-20-15										
#6 Leg curl	4	12-10-10-8										
#7 Dumbbell lunges	4	12-10-10-8										
#8 Leg Ups	4	18-16-14-12										
#9 Shoulder shrug (optional)	4	12-10-10-8										
Friday - Arms, Quads and Abs'												
#1 Cambered bar (crooked bar) standing curls	4	12-10-10-8										
#2 Seated overhead triceps extension	4	12-10-10-8										
#3 Dumbbell incline bench rotating biceps curl	4	12-10-10-8										
#4 V-Bar press downs	4	12-10-10-8										
#5 Hammer Curls	4	12-10-10-8										
#6 Reverse grip straight bar extensions	4	12-10-10-8										
#7 Leg extension	4	12-10-10-8										
#8 Dumbbell lunges	4	12-10-10-8										
#9 Leg Ups	4	18-16-14-12										
#10 Crunch on the floor (really try to feel the squeeze)	4	30-25-20-15										

*First set is always a warm up

Michael S. Kamins

Appendix 5 EXERCISE CHART – 8 Week (copy and use for your own, or email me for the Excel file)

8 WEEK PROGRAM	Sets*	Reps	Week 1 (date)	Week 2 (date)	Week 3 (date)	Week 4 (date)	Week 5 (date)	Week 6 (date)	Week 7 (date)	Week 8 (date)
Monday - Chest and Calves										
#1 Incline dumbbell chest press	4	12-10-10-8								
#2 Standing calf raises (biggest text book or step)	4	30-25-20-15								
#3 Flat bench dumbbell press	4	12-10-10-8								
#4 Weighted calf raise	4	16-14-12-10								
#5 Dumbbell Flyes	4	12-10-10-8								
#6 Pushups (no warm up)	3	12 to 15								
Tuesday - Back and Abs										
#1 Wide grip pull down	4	12-10-10-8								
#2 One arm dumbbell row	4	12-10-10-8								
#3 Leg Ups	4	12-10-10-8								
#4 Crunch on the floor	4	30-25-20-15								
#5 Narrow grip pull downs	4	12-10-10-8								
#6 Reverse grip pull downs	4	12-10-10-8								
Wednesday - Hamstrings and Quads										
#1 Dumbbell Squat	4	12-10-10-8								
#2 Leg extension	4	12-10-10-8								
#3 Dumbbell lunges	4	12-10-10-8								
#4 Leg curl	4	12-10-10-8								
Thursday - Shoulders, Calves and Traps										
#1 Dumbbell press	4	12-10-10-8								
#2 Dumbbell rear shoulder raise	4	12-10-10-8								
#3 Standing calf (biggest textbook or step)	4	30-25-20-15								
#4 Dumbbell shoulder shrug	4	12-10-10-8								
#5 Upright rows	4	12-10-10-8								
#6 Weighted calf raise	4	16-14-12-10								
#7 Dumbbell forward shoulder raise	4	20-10-10-8								
#8 Toes out calves raises	4	20-18-16-14								
Friday - Arms and Abs										
#1 Leg Ups	4	18-16-14-12								
#2 Cambered bar (crooked bar) standing curls	4	12-10-10-8								
#3 Seated overhead triceps extension	4	12-10-10-8								
#4 Dumbbell incline bench rotating biceps curl	4	12-10-10-8								
#5 V-Bar press downs	4	12-10-10-8								
#6 Crunch on the floor (really try to feel the squeeze)	4	30-25-20-15								
#7 Hammer Curls	4	12-10-10-8								
#8 Reverse grip straight bar extensions	4	12-10-10-8								

*First set is always a warm up(except for push ups)